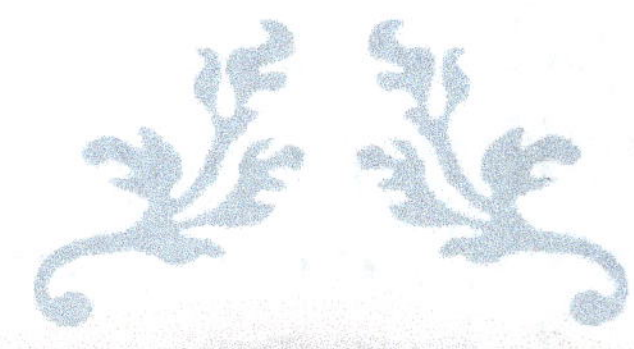

THE COMPLETE LYMPHATIC DIET COOKBOOK 2024

Easy and Delicious Recipes including health benefits, meal plan and portion control

MICHAEL L. ALLEN

TABLE OF CONTENTS

Introduction

Welcome to the world of the Lymphatic Diet, where wellness meets science in optimizing your body's natural detoxification system. Unlike fad diets that promise quick fixes, the Lymphatic Diet focuses on nurturing your lymphatic system, a vital but often overlooked component of your body's immune and waste elimination processes.

In this exclusive content, we'll dive into the fundamentals of the Lymphatic Diet, exploring how it works, its benefits, and practical steps to incorporate it into your lifestyle seamlessly.

But first, let's understand the role of the lymphatic system. Think of it as your body's internal sanitation department, responsible for removing toxins, waste products, and excess fluids from your tissues. When the lymphatic system is functioning optimally, you feel energized, vibrant, and resilient to illnesses. However, factors like poor diet, sedentary lifestyle, stress, and environmental toxins can impede its efficiency, leading to symptoms like bloating, fatigue, and weakened immunity.

The Lymphatic Diet aims to support and enhance your lymphatic system's function through nourishing foods, hydration, movement, and stress management. By prioritizing foods rich in antioxidants, anti-inflammatory compounds, and essential nutrients, you provide your body with the building blocks it needs to maintain a healthy lymphatic system.

In the upcoming sections, we'll explore specific dietary recommendations, lifestyle practices, and recipes designed to promote lymphatic health and overall well-being. Whether you're looking to boost your energy levels, improve digestion, or support your body's natural detoxification process, the Lymphatic Diet offers a holistic approach to health and vitality.

Get ready to embark on a journey towards better health and vitality as we uncover the transformative power of the Lymphatic Diet. Let's nourish, cleanse, and revitalize our bodies from the inside out.

BENEFITS OF THE LYMPHATIC DIET

Detoxification and Immune Support:

The lymphatic system plays a pivotal role in detoxification and immune function. The lymphatic diet focuses on consuming foods that support

lymphatic circulation and drainage, such as fresh fruits, vegetables, and herbs. These nutrient-rich foods provide antioxidants, vitamins, and minerals essential for neutralizing toxins and strengthening the immune system. By following a lymphatic diet, individuals can enhance detoxification processes and bolster their body's natural defenses against infections and diseases.

Reduced Inflammation:

Numerous medical diseases, such as autoimmune disorders, cardiovascular disease, and arthritis, are associated with chronic inflammation. The lymphatic diet emphasizes anti-inflammatory foods like leafy greens, berries, fatty fish, and nuts, which help reduce inflammation throughout the body. By adopting this dietary approach, individuals can potentially alleviate symptoms associated with inflammation and promote overall wellness.

Weight Management:

For general health and longevity, it is essential to maintain a healthy weight. The lymphatic diet encourages the consumption of whole, nutrient-dense foods while limiting processed foods, refined sugars, and unhealthy fats. This approach supports sustainable weight management by promoting satiety, stabilizing blood sugar levels, and enhancing metabolism. Additionally, by improving lymphatic circulation and reducing inflammation, the lymphatic diet may aid in shedding excess pounds and achieving a healthier body composition.

Enhanced Digestive Health:

A well-functioning lymphatic system is essential for optimal digestive health. The lymphatic diet includes foods rich in fiber, probiotics, and digestive enzymes, which support gastrointestinal function and promote regularity. Incorporating fermented foods like yogurt, kimchi, and sauerkraut can help maintain a healthy balance of gut bacteria, improve nutrient absorption, and reduce the risk of digestive issues such as bloating, constipation, and irritable bowel syndrome (IBS).

Skin Health and Beauty:

The health of the lymphatic system is closely tied to the appearance of the skin. Congestion in the lymphatic system can manifest as dull, congested skin, acne, and puffiness. By following a lymphatic diet rich in hydrating foods, antioxidants, and essential fatty acids, individuals can nourish their skin from within, promoting a radiant complexion and youthful appearance. Furthermore, by supporting lymphatic drainage and circulation, the lymphatic diet may help reduce the appearance of cellulite and promote skin elasticity and tone.

THE LYMPHATIC DIET FOR OPTIMAL HEALTH

Understanding the Lymphatic System:

The lymphatic system is a network of vessels and organs that help eliminate toxins, waste, and excess fluid from the body. It also plays a vital role in immune function by transporting white blood cells throughout the body to fight off infections and diseases.

Key Principles of the Lymphatic Diet:

- **Hydration:** Adequate hydration is essential for maintaining lymphatic flow. Drink plenty of water throughout the day to keep the lymphatic system functioning optimally.
- **Whole Foods:** Focus on consuming whole, nutrient-dense foods such as fruits, vegetables, whole grains, and lean proteins. These foods provide essential vitamins, minerals, and antioxidants that support lymphatic health.
- **Limit Processed Foods:** Processed foods, high in sugar, unhealthy fats, and artificial additives, can contribute to inflammation and hinder lymphatic function. Limit your intake of processed foods and opt for whole food alternatives whenever possible.
- **Incorporate Lymphatic-Friendly Foods:** Certain foods are particularly beneficial for promoting lymphatic flow, including citrus fruits, leafy greens, berries, garlic, ginger, turmeric, and omega-3 fatty

acids found in fatty fish and flaxseeds.

- **Herbal Support:** Herbal teas such as dandelion root, cleavers, and echinacea can help support lymphatic function and detoxification.
- **Exercise Regularly:** Regular physical activity, such as walking, yoga, rebounding, or swimming, can stimulate lymphatic circulation and promote detoxification.
- **Lymphatic Massage:** Consider incorporating lymphatic massage techniques into your self-care routine to help stimulate lymphatic flow and reduce fluid retention.
- **Manage Stress:** Chronic stress can impair lymphatic function and weaken the immune system. Practice stress-reducing techniques such as meditation, deep breathing exercises, or mindfulness to support overall well-being.

ESSENTIAL INGREDIENTS AND COOKING TIPS

Essential Ingredients:

- Leafy Greens: Incorporate an abundance of leafy greens like spinach, kale, and Swiss chard into your meals. These greens are rich in chlorophyll, antioxidants, and fiber, which help to cleanse the lymphatic system and promote detoxification.

- Citrus Fruits: Citrus fruits such as lemons, oranges, and grapefruits are excellent sources of vitamin C and antioxidants. These nutrients support lymphatic function by reducing inflammation and boosting immune health.

- **Berries:** Berries like blueberries, strawberries, and raspberries are packed with antioxidants called flavonoids, which help to protect lymphatic vessels from damage and improve circulation.

- **Cruciferous Vegetables:** Broccoli, cauliflower, and Brussels sprouts are part of the cruciferous vegetable family, known for their detoxifying properties. These veggies contain compounds like sulforaphane, which supports lymphatic health by aiding in the elimination of toxins.

- **Omega-3 Rich Foods:** Include omega-3 fatty acids from sources like salmon, walnuts, and flaxseeds in your diet. Omega-3s help to reduce inflammation in the body, which can benefit lymphatic function.

Cooking Tips:

- Steam or Saute: Opt for cooking methods like steaming or sautéing rather than trying to preserve the nutritional value of your ingredients. These methods retain more nutrients and reduce the intake of unhealthy fats that can impair lymphatic function.
- **Use Herbs and Spices:** Incorporate herbs and spices like turmeric, ginger, garlic, and cilantro into your cooking. These ingredients have anti-inflammatory and detoxifying properties that support lymphatic health.

- **Drink A Lot of Water:** Throughout the day, make sure you stay hydrated by drinking a lot of water. Proper hydration is essential for lymphatic circulation and helps to flush out toxins from the body.
- **Limit Processed Foods:** Minimize your intake of processed foods, refined sugars, and unhealthy fats, as these can contribute to inflammation and lymphatic congestion. Focus on whole, nutrient-dense foods instead.
- **Practice Mindful Eating:** Take the time to savor and enjoy your meals, and pay attention to how different foods make you feel. Mindful eating can help you tune into your body's signals and make healthier choices that support lymphatic function.

1

Breakfast Recipes

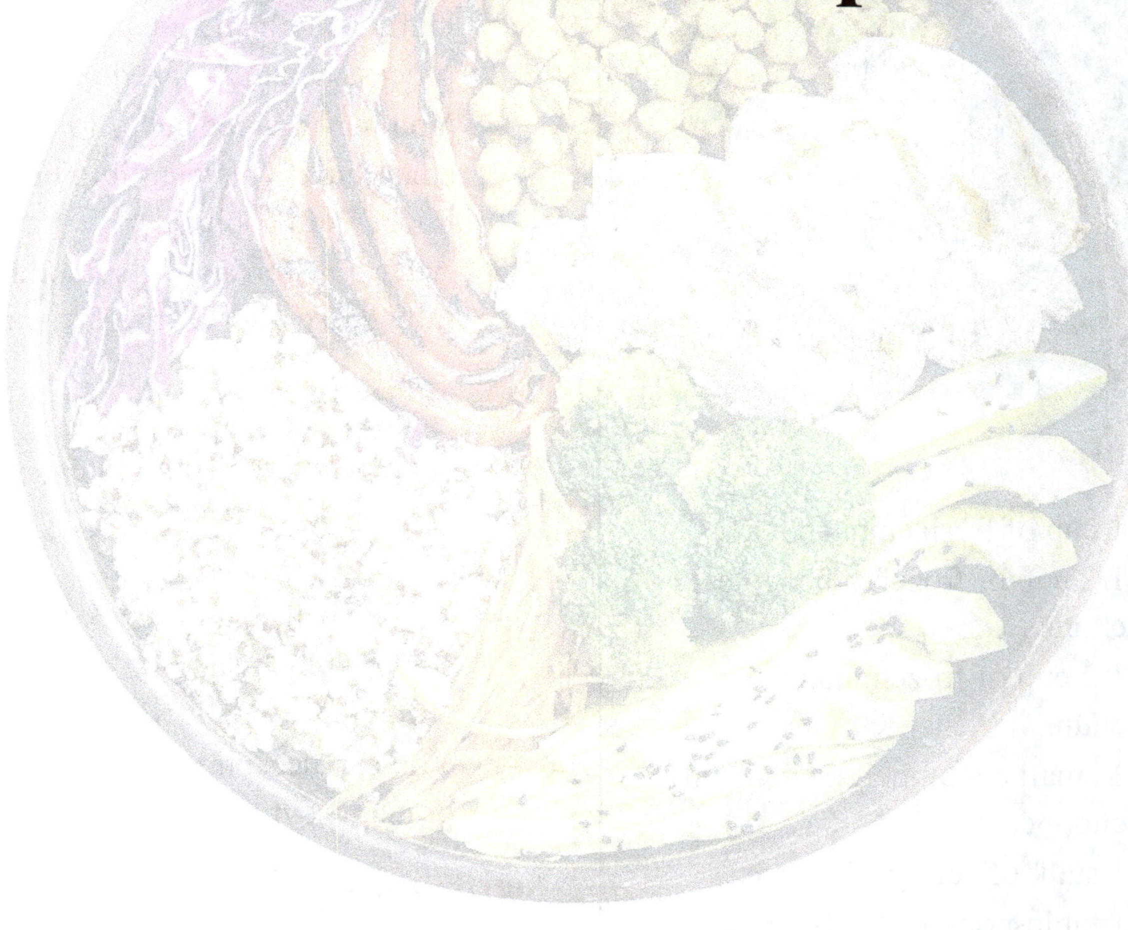

LYMPHATIC BOOSTING SMOOTHIE

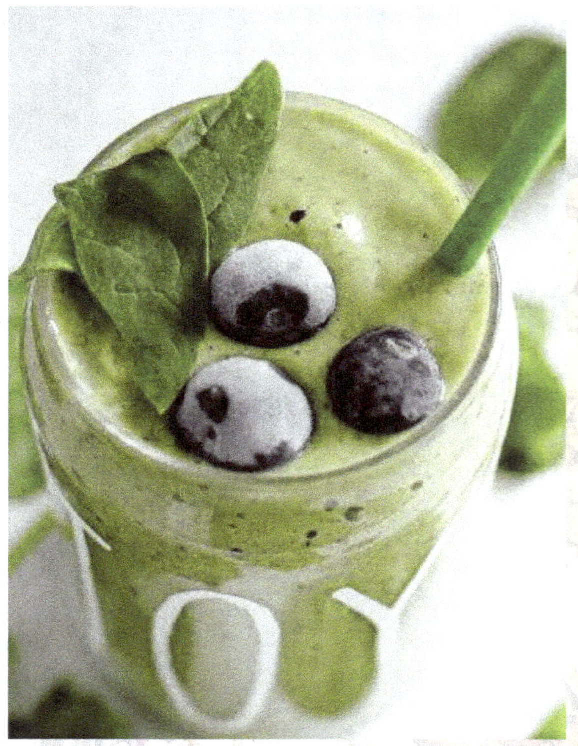

Ingredients

- 1 cup of fresh spinach leaves
- 1/2 cup of frozen pineapple chunks
- 1/2 cup of frozen mango chunks
- 1 small cucumber, peeled and chopped
- 1 stalk of celery, chopped
- 1 tablespoon of fresh ginger, grated
- 1 tablespoon of chia seeds
- 1 tablespoon of lemon juice
- 1 cup of coconut water
- Ice cubes (optional)

Procedure

- Wash all the fresh produce thoroughly.
- In a blender, combine the spinach, pineapple chunks, mango chunks, cucumber, celery, ginger, chia seeds, lemon juice, and coconut water.
- Until smooth and creamy, process at a high speed.
- You may add ice cubes to the smoothie if you want it to be thicker and cooler.
- After transferring the smoothie into glasses, serve it right away.

Time of Preparation

- Approximately 10 minutes

Tips and Tricks

- You can change the smoothie's consistency by adding or removing coconut water.
- You can use a tiny bit of honey or maple syrup for sweetness.

Nutritional Value per Serving

- **Calories: 120**
- **Protein: 3g**
- **Carbohydrates: 25g**
- **Fat: 2g**

- **Fiber: 7g**
- **Vitamin C: 70% DV**
- **Vitamin A: 80% DV**
- **Iron: 10% DV**
- **Calcium: 8% DV**

Caution and Precautions

- If you have any allergies to the ingredients listed, avoid consuming this smoothie.
- Consult with a healthcare professional if you have any medical conditions or concerns about incorporating this smoothie into your diet.
- Be cautious when using ginger, especially if you are pregnant or have digestive issues, as it can cause discomfort in some individuals.

Health Benefits of this Recipe

- Supports lymphatic system function: The combination of spinach, cucumber, celery, and ginger in this smoothie contains compounds that can help promote lymphatic drainage and circulation, aiding in detoxification and immune function.
- Rich in antioxidants: Pineapple, mango, and spinach are all rich sources of antioxidants such as vitamin C and beta-carotene, which help protect cells from damage caused by free radicals.
- Hydration: Coconut water provides electrolytes and hydration, making this smoothie a refreshing and hydrating option, especially after exercise or during hot weather.
- Digestive support: Chia seeds are high in fiber, which can promote healthy digestion and regular bowel movements.

Healthy Safety Measures

- Wash your hands and all utensils thoroughly before preparing the smoothie to avoid contamination.
- Use a clean cutting board and knife to chop the fruits and vegetables.
- Store any leftover smoothie in an airtight container in the refrigerator for up to 24 hours to maintain freshness and prevent bacterial growth.

QUINOA BREAKFAST BOWL

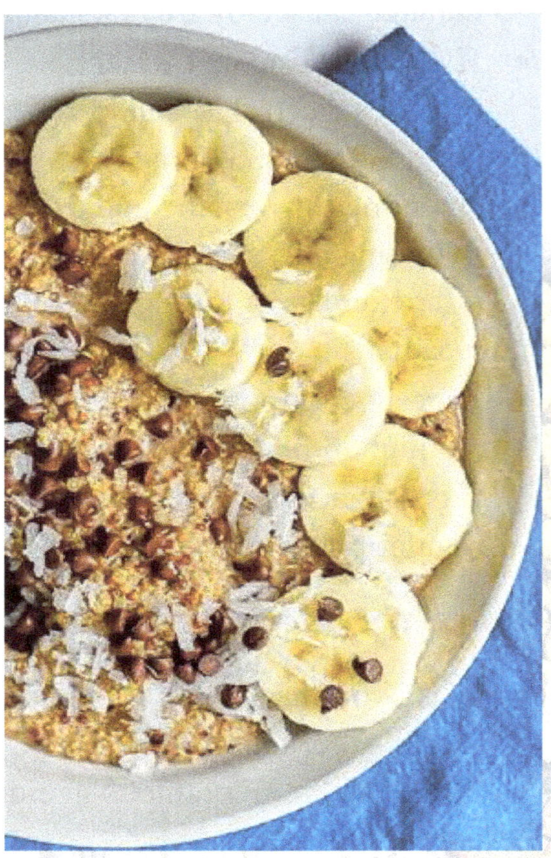

Ingredients

- 1/2 cup quinoa, rinsed
- 1 cup water or almond milk
- 1 tablespoon maple syrup or honey (optional)
- 1/2 teaspoon cinnamon
- Half a cup of mixed berries, including raspberries, blueberries, and strawberries
- 1/4 cup sliced almonds or walnuts
- 1 ripe banana, sliced
- 1 tablespoon chia seeds
- Greek yogurt or coconut yogurt for topping (optional)

Procedure

- In a small saucepan, combine the quinoa and water (or almond milk) and bring to a boil.
- Once the quinoa is cooked and the liquid has been absorbed, reduce the heat to low, cover, and simmer for 15 to 20 minutes.
- Stir in the maple syrup (or honey) and cinnamon.
- Divide the cooked quinoa into serving bowls.
- Top each bowl with mixed berries, sliced almonds (or walnuts), sliced banana, and chia seeds.
- If desired, add a dollop of Greek yogurt or coconut yogurt on top for extra creaminess.

Time of Preparation

- Approximately 25 minutes

Tips and Tricks

- Rinse the quinoa before cooking to remove any bitter coating called saponin.
- For a creamier texture, cook the quinoa in almond milk instead of water.
- Customize your breakfast bowl with your favorite toppings such as sliced peaches,

shredded coconut, or a drizzle of nut butter.

- Make a batch of quinoa ahead of time and store it in the refrigerator for quick and easy breakfasts throughout the week.

Nutritional Value per Serving

- **Calories: 350**
- **Protein: 10g**
- **Carbohydrates: 55g**
- **Fat: 10g**
- **Fiber: 8g**
- **Vitamin C: 15% DV**
- **Calcium: 10% DV**
- **Iron: 20% DV**

Caution and Precautions

- Check the quinoa for any debris before rinsing to ensure it's clean.
- Be cautious when adding sweeteners like maple syrup or honey, especially if you are watching your sugar intake.
- If you have a nut allergy, omit the sliced almonds or walnuts and choose a different topping option.

Health Benefits of this Recipe

- High in protein: Quinoa is a great option for vegetarians and vegans as it is a complete protein, meaning it includes all nine essential amino acids.
- Rich in fiber: Quinoa and chia seeds are both high in fiber, which can promote digestive health and keep you feeling full and satisfied throughout the morning.
- Antioxidant-rich: Berries are packed with antioxidants, vitamins, and minerals that help protect cells from damage caused by free radicals and support overall health.
- Heart-healthy fats: Almonds and walnuts are rich in heart-healthy fats, such as omega-3 fatty acids, which can help reduce inflammation and lower the risk of heart disease.

Healthy Safety Measures

- To avoid cross-contamination, use different cutting boards and tools for raw fruits and vegetables.
- Store leftover quinoa breakfast bowls in airtight containers in the refrigerator for up to 3-4 days.
- Reheat leftovers thoroughly before consuming to reduce the risk of foodborne illness.

GREEN DETOX JUICE

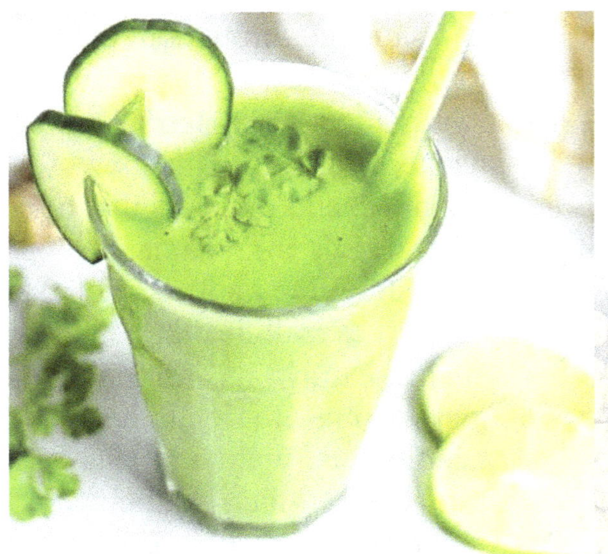

Ingredients

- 2 cups spinach leaves
- 1 cucumber, peeled and chopped
- 2 stalks celery, chopped
- 1 green apple, cored and chopped
- 1/2 lemon, peeled
- 1-inch piece of ginger, peeled
- 1 tablespoon fresh parsley leaves (optional)
- 1 cup water
- Ice cubes (optional)

Procedure

- Wash all the fresh produce thoroughly.
- In a juicer or blender, combine the spinach leaves, cucumber, celery, green apple, lemon, ginger, and parsley leaves (if using).
- Add water to help with blending.
- Blend or juice until smooth.
- If desired, remove pulp from the mixture by straining it through cheesecloth or a fine mesh sieve
- If desired, pour the juice into glasses with ice cubes in them.
- Serve immediately and enjoy!

Time of Preparation

- Approximately 10 minutes

Tips and Tricks

- When feasible, use organic, fresh ingredients for the greatest taste and nutritious content.
- Adjust the ingredients to suit your taste preferences. You can add more apple for sweetness or more lemon for acidity.
- If using a blender, you may need to add more water to help with blending, and you may want to strain the mixture to remove pulp for a smoother juice.

- For added freshness, serve the juice immediately after preparing.

Nutritional Value per Serving

- **Calories: 70**
- **Protein: 2g**
- **Carbohydrates: 17g**
- **Fat: 0.5g**
- **Fiber: 4g**
- **Vitamin C: 60% DV**
- **Vitamin A: 90% DV**
- **Iron: 10% DV**
- **Calcium: 8% DV**

Caution and Precautions

- Be cautious when consuming large quantities of green juice, as it can be high in natural sugars from the fruits, which may affect blood sugar levels.
- If you have any medical conditions or concerns, consult with a healthcare professional before incorporating this juice into your diet.
- Avoid using too much ginger if you are sensitive to its spicy flavor or if you have gastrointestinal issues.

Health Benefits of this Recipe

- Detoxifying properties: The combination of spinach, cucumber, celery, lemon, and ginger in this juice helps support the body's natural detoxification process by flushing out toxins and promoting healthy digestion.
- Nutrient-rich: This juice is packed with vitamins, minerals, and antioxidants from the green vegetables and fruits, which support overall health and well-being.
- Hydration: Cucumber and lemon are high in water content, helping to keep you hydrated and refreshed.
- Anti-inflammatory: Ginger contains bioactive compounds that have anti-inflammatory properties, which may help reduce inflammation and support immune function.

Healthy Safety Measures

- Wash your hands and all utensils thoroughly before preparing the juice to avoid contamination.
- Clean the juicer or blender thoroughly after each use to prevent bacterial growth.

- Store any leftover juice in an airtight container in the refrigerator for up to 24 hours

to maintain freshness and prevent spoilage

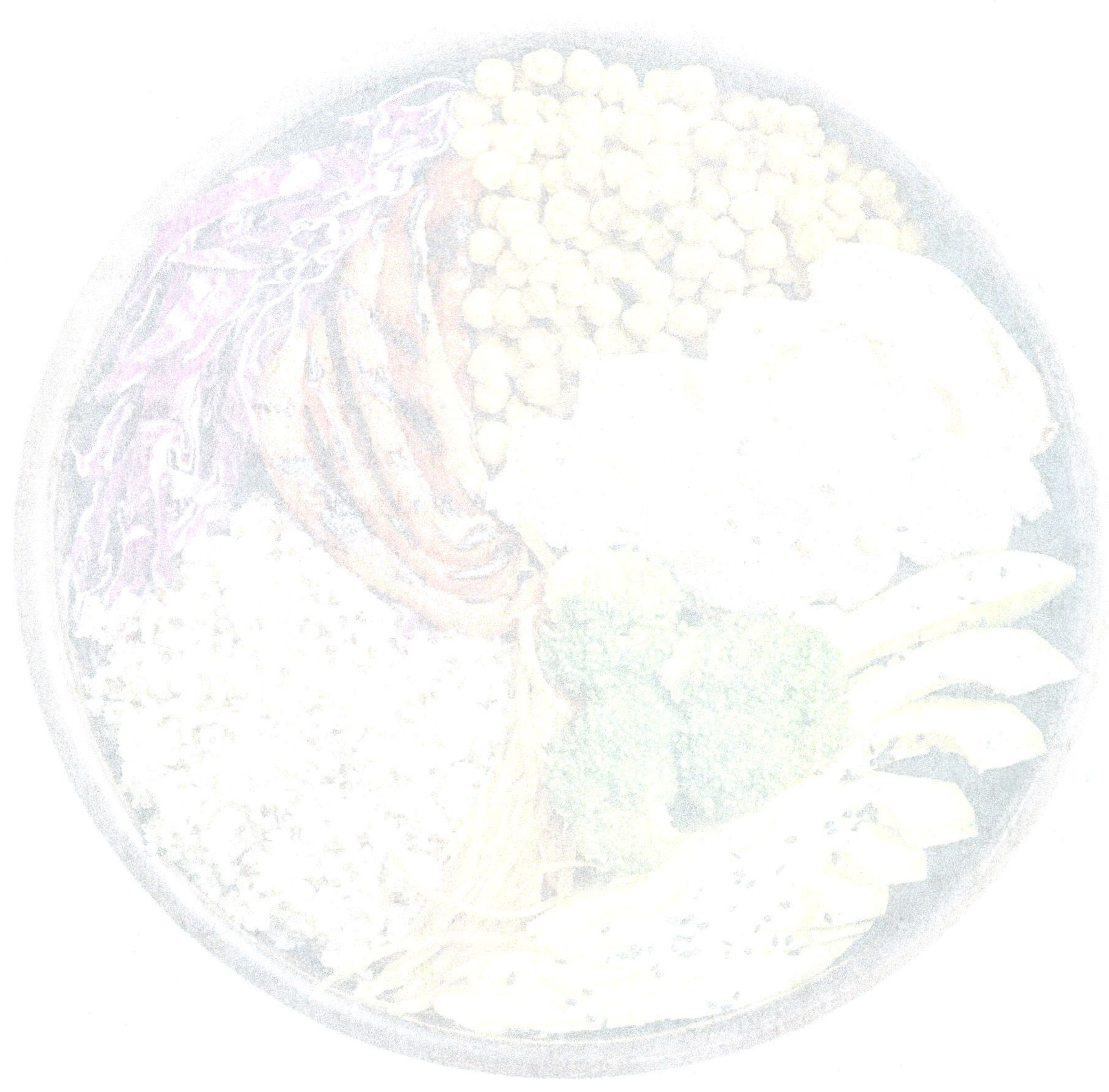

2

Lunch Recipes

Lymphatic Cleansing Salad

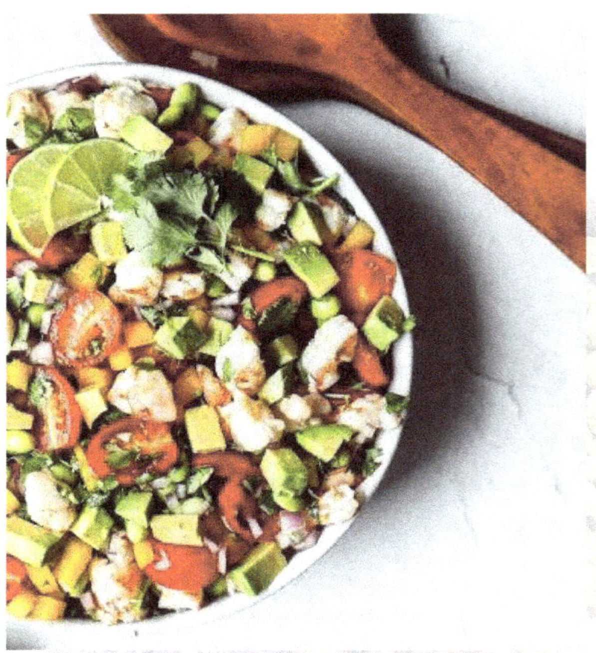

Ingredients

- 2 cups mixed greens (such as spinach, kale, and arugula)
- 1 cup chopped cucumber
- 1 cup diced bell peppers (assorted colors)
- 1 cup cherry tomatoes, halved
- ½ cup shredded carrots
- ¼ cup chopped fresh parsley
- ¼ cup chopped fresh cilantro
- 2 tablespoons extra virgin olive oil
- 1 tablespoon freshly squeezed lemon juice
- 1 teaspoon raw apple cider vinegar
- 1 clove garlic, minced
- Salt and pepper to taste

Procedure

- Wash all vegetables thoroughly under running water and pat them dry.
- In a large mixing bowl, combine the mixed greens, cucumber, bell peppers, cherry tomatoes, shredded carrots, parsley, and cilantro.
- In a small bowl, whisk together the olive oil, lemon juice, apple cider vinegar, minced garlic, salt, and pepper to make the dressing.
- After adding the dressing to the salad, carefully toss everything to coat.
- Serve immediately as a refreshing and cleansing meal.

Time of Preparation

- Approximately 15 minutes

Tips and Tricks

- Use fresh and organic ingredients whenever possible to maximize the nutritional value of the salad.
- Feel free to customize the salad with your favorite vegetables or add protein sources like grilled chicken or tofu for a more satisfying meal.
- For added flavor, you can sprinkle some toasted nuts or

seeds on top of the salad before serving.

Nutritional Value per Serving

- **Calories: 120**
- **Total Fat: 8g**
- **Saturated Fat: 1g**
- **Cholesterol: 0mg**
- **Sodium: 50mg**
- **Total Carbohydrates: 12g**
- **Dietary Fiber: 4g**
- **Sugars: 5g**
- **Protein: 3g**

Caution and Precautions

- If you have any allergies or sensitivities to certain ingredients, be sure to omit or substitute them accordingly.
- Always consult with a healthcare professional before making significant changes to your diet, especially if you have any underlying health conditions or concerns.

Health Benefits of this Recipe

- Rich in fiber: The combination of vegetables in this salad provides a good amount of dietary fiber, which promotes healthy digestion and regular bowel movements.
- Antioxidant-rich: The colorful array of vegetables in this salad is packed with antioxidants that help protect cells from damage caused by free radicals and support overall health.
- Hydrating: Cucumber and tomatoes are high in water content, helping to keep you hydrated and maintain optimal fluid balance in the body.
- Supports detoxification: Ingredients like parsley and cilantro are known for their detoxifying properties, helping to support the body's natural detoxification processes, including lymphatic drainage.

Healthy Safety Measures

- Wash your hands thoroughly before handling food to prevent the spread of bacteria and contaminants.
- Use separate cutting boards and utensils for raw vegetables and other ingredients to avoid cross-contamination.
- Store leftovers in an airtight container in the refrigerator and consume within 1-2 days to maintain freshness and prevent foodborne illness.

LENTIL SOUP WITH TURMERIC

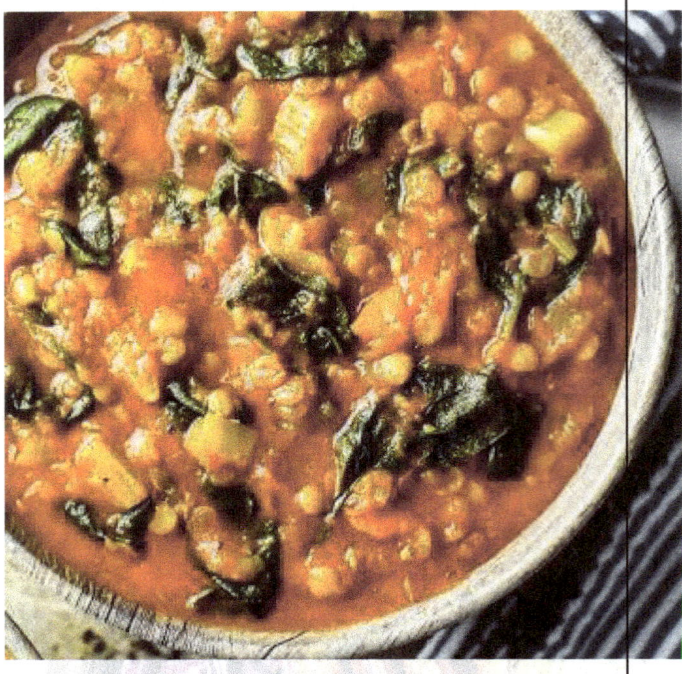

Ingredients

- 1 cup dried lentils, rinsed and drained
- 4 cups vegetable broth
- 1 onion, finely chopped
- 2 carrots, diced
- 2 celery stalks, diced
- 3 cloves garlic, minced
- 1 tablespoon olive oil
- 1 teaspoon ground turmeric
- 1 teaspoon ground cumin
- ½ teaspoon ground coriander
- ¼ teaspoon ground ginger
- Salt and pepper to taste
- Fresh cilantro or parsley for garnish (optional)

Procedure

- In a large pot, heat the olive oil over medium heat. Cook the chopped onion, carrots, and celery for five to seven minutes, or until they are tender.
- Add the minced garlic, turmeric, cumin, coriander, and ginger to the pot, and cook for another minute until fragrant.
- Add the rinsed lentils and vegetable broth to the pot, and bring to a boil.
- Once the lentils are soft, reduce the heat to low, cover, and simmer for 20 to 25 minutes.
- Adjust the seasoning with salt and pepper to taste.
- If preferred, top with freshly chopped parsley or cilantro and serve hot.

Time of Preparation

- Approximately 35-40 minutes

Tips and Tricks

- Instead of using dried lentils, you can use canned lentils to save time. Toss them into the soup after giving them a quick rinse and drain.
- For extra flavor, you can sauté the spices with the vegetables before adding the broth and lentils.
- Feel free to add other vegetables like spinach, kale, or tomatoes to the soup for added nutrition and flavor.

Nutritional Value per Serving

- **Calories: 200**
- **Total Fat: 3g**
- **Saturated Fat: 0.5g**
- **Cholesterol: 0mg**
- **Sodium: 600mg**
- **Total Carbohydrates: 35g**
- **Dietary Fiber: 15g**
- **Sugars: 5g**
- **Protein: 13g**

Caution and Precautions

- Be cautious when handling turmeric, as it can stain surfaces and clothing.
- If you are taking any medications or have a medical condition, consult with your healthcare provider before consuming turmeric regularly, as it may interact with certain medications or exacerbate certain health conditions.

Health Benefits of this Recipe

- Rich in fiber: Lentils are an excellent source of dietary fiber, which helps promote digestive health and regulate blood sugar levels.
- Anti-inflammatory properties: Turmeric contains curcumin, a compound known for its powerful anti-inflammatory and antioxidant properties, which may help reduce inflammation and protect against chronic diseases.
- Heart-healthy: Lentils are low in fat and cholesterol and high in potassium, which can help lower blood pressure and reduce the risk of heart disease.
- Immune-boosting: The combination of vegetables and spices in this soup provides essential vitamins, minerals, and antioxidants that support a healthy immune system.

Healthy Safety Measures

- Wash your hands thoroughly before and after handling raw ingredients to prevent the spread of bacteria.
- Use separate cutting boards and utensils for raw vegetables and other ingredients to avoid cross-contamination.
- Store leftover soup in an airtight container in the refrigerator and consume within 3-4 days to maintain freshness and prevent foodborne illness.

GRILLED VEGETABLE WRAP

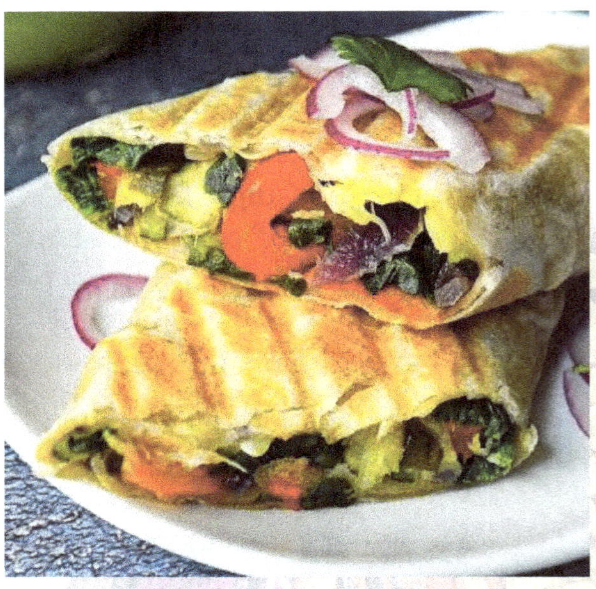

Ingredients

- 1 large whole wheat or spinach tortilla wrap
- 1 zucchini, sliced lengthwise
- 1 yellow squash, sliced lengthwise
- 1 red bell pepper, sliced
- 1 yellow bell pepper, sliced
- 1 small eggplant, sliced into rounds
- 1 tablespoon olive oil
- 1 teaspoon Italian seasoning
- Salt and pepper to taste
- Hummus or tzatziki sauce for spreading
- Fresh spinach leaves or mixed greens for filling
- Optional additional fillings: sliced avocado, shredded carrots, diced tomatoes, feta cheese

Procedure

- Turn the heat up to medium-high on the grill or grill pan.
- In a large bowl, toss the sliced zucchini, yellow squash, bell peppers, and eggplant with olive oil, Italian seasoning, salt, and pepper until evenly coated.
- Place the vegetables on the grill and cook for 3-4 minutes per side, or until they are tender and have grill marks.
- After grilling, take the veggies off of the grill and place them aside.
- Warm the tortilla wrap on the grill for about 30 seconds on each side, or until it is pliable.
- Spread a layer of hummus or tzatziki sauce onto the center of the tortilla wrap.
- Arrange the grilled vegetables and any additional fillings you desire on top of the sauce.
- Add a handful of fresh spinach leaves or mixed greens on top of the vegetables.

- Fold in the sides of the tortilla, then roll it up tightly from the bottom to enclose the filling.
- Cut the wrapper in half on the diagonal and start serving right away.

Time of Preparation

- Approximately 20-25 minutes

Tips and Tricks

- To prevent the vegetables from sticking to the grill, lightly brush them with olive oil before grilling.
- You can use a grill basket or skewers to grill smaller or more delicate vegetables like cherry tomatoes or mushrooms.
- If you don't have a grill, you can roast the vegetables in the oven at 400°F (200°C) for about 20 minutes, or until they are tender.

Nutritional Value per Serving

- Calories: 250
- Total Fat: 10g
- Saturated Fat: 1.5g
- Cholesterol: 0mg
- Sodium: 350mg
- Total Carbohydrates: 35g
- Dietary Fiber: 8g
- Sugars: 5g

- Protein: 7g

Caution and Precautions

- Be careful when handling hot grilling equipment to avoid burns or injuries.
- Make sure the grill or grill pan is properly cleaned and preheated before cooking to ensure even cooking and prevent foodborne illness.

Health Benefits of this Recipe

- Rich in vitamins and minerals: Grilled vegetables are packed with essential nutrients like vitamins A, C, and K, as well as potassium and fiber, which are important for overall health and well-being.
- Low in calories and fat: This wrap is a light and satisfying meal option that is low in calories and fat, making it suitable for those looking to maintain a healthy weight or reduce their calorie intake.
- Plant-based protein: Hummus or tzatziki sauce adds a creamy texture and a boost of protein to the wrap, making it a filling and nutritious option for vegetarians and vegans.

- Heart-healthy: The combination of whole wheat tortilla, grilled vegetables, and healthy fats from olive oil provides heart-healthy nutrients that can help lower cholesterol levels and reduce the risk of heart disease.

Healthy Safety Measures

- Wash your hands thoroughly before and after handling raw vegetables to prevent the spread of bacteria.
- Clean and sanitize grilling equipment and surfaces regularly to prevent cross-contamination and foodborne illness.
- Store leftover grilled vegetables and wrap components in separate airtight containers in the refrigerator and consume within 2-3 days to maintain freshness and prevent spoilage.

3

Dinner Recipes

GARLIC GINGER SALMON

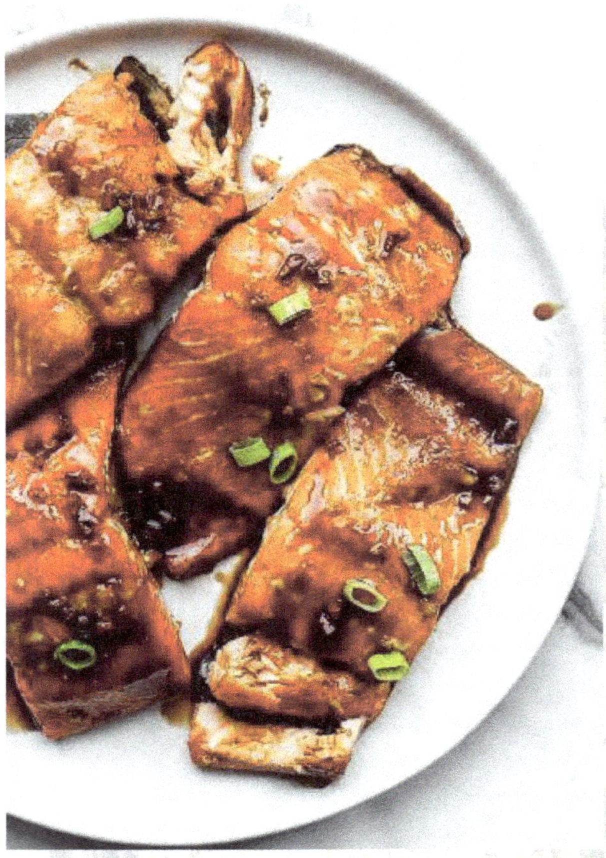

Ingredients

- 4 salmon fillets
- 4 cloves garlic, minced
- 2 tablespoons grated ginger
- 1/4 cup soy sauce
- 2 tablespoons honey
- 2 tablespoons olive oil
- 1 tablespoon rice vinegar
- 1 tablespoon sesame oil
- Salt and pepper to taste
- Sesame seeds and sliced green onions as garnish

Procedure

- Preparation: Preheat the oven to 400°F (200°C). For easier cleanup, line a baking pan with aluminum foil or parchment paper.
- Marinade: In a small bowl, whisk together the minced garlic, grated ginger, soy sauce, honey, olive oil, rice vinegar, sesame oil, salt, and pepper.
- To marinate salmon, put the fillets in a plastic bag that can be sealed tightly or in a shallow dish. Make sure all of the salmon fillets are equally coated when you pour the marinade over them. Let it marinate in the fridge for a minimum of half an hour, or for maximum flavor, up to two hours.
- Cooking: Remove the salmon from the marinade and place them on the prepared baking sheet. Discard any leftover marinade. For 12 to 15 minutes, or until the salmon flakes easily with a fork, bake it in the preheated oven.
- Garnish: Once cooked, remove the salmon from the oven and

garnish with sliced green onions and sesame seeds for added flavor and presentation.

Time of Preparation

- Approximately 45 minutes (including marinating time).

Tips and Tricks

- For extra flavor, you can add a splash of lemon juice to the marinade.
- Make sure to not overcook the salmon to keep it moist and tender. Once cooked, it ought to flake easily with a fork.
- If you prefer a stronger ginger flavor, you can increase the amount of grated ginger in the marinade.

Nutritional Value per Serving

- **Calories: 300 kcal**
- **Protein: 25g**
- **Fat: 18g**
- **Carbohydrates: 9g**
- **Fiber: 1g**
- **Sugar: 7g**

Caution and Precautions

- Be careful when handling raw salmon to avoid cross-contamination with other foods.

After handling, properly wash your hands and any surfaces.
- Ensure the salmon reaches an internal temperature of at least 145°F (63°C) to ensure it is safe to eat.

Health Benefits of this Recipe

- Omega-3 fatty acids, which are abundant in salmon, have been shown to lower inflammation and promote heart health.
- Garlic and ginger are known for their immune-boosting properties and can help fight off infections.
- The marinade contains minimal added sugars and unhealthy fats, making this recipe a healthier option compared to fried or heavily processed dishes.

Healthy Safety Measures

- Use fresh salmon fillets from a reputable source to ensure quality and safety.
- Wash hands and utensils thoroughly before and after handling raw ingredients to prevent contamination.
- Store leftovers in an airtight container in the refrigerator and consume within 2-3 days.

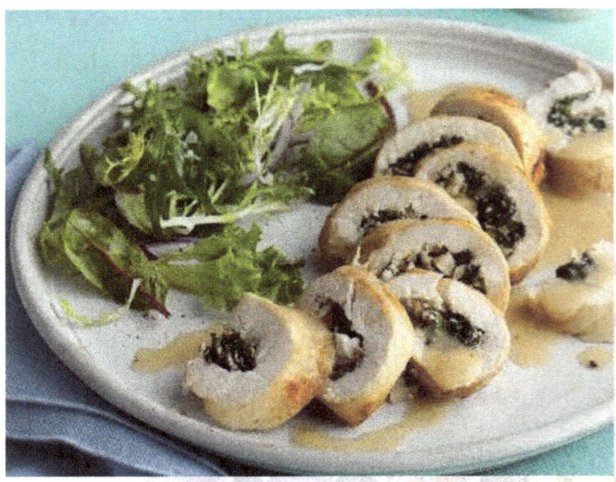

Ingredients

- 4 boneless, skinless chicken breasts
- 2 cups fresh spinach, chopped
- 1 cup mushrooms, sliced
- 1/2 cup shredded mozzarella cheese
- 2 cloves garlic, minced
- 1 tablespoon olive oil
- 1 teaspoon Italian seasoning
- Salt and pepper to taste
- Toothpicks or kitchen twine for securing the chicken

Procedure

- Preparation: Preheat the oven to 375°F (190°C). Use non-stick cooking spray or olive oil to grease a baking dish.
- To prepare the filling, heat up some olive oil in a skillet over medium heat. Add the minced garlic and simmer for one minute, or until fragrant. Add sliced mushrooms and cook until they are tender and browned, about 5-7 minutes. Add chopped spinach and cook until wilted. Season with salt, pepper, and Italian seasoning. Take off the heat and allow to cool a little.
- Butterfly the Chicken: Lay each chicken breast flat on a cutting board. With a sharp knife, carefully slice horizontally through the thickest part of the chicken breast, stopping about 1/2 inch from the edge, to create a pocket for the filling.
- Stuffing the Chicken: Divide the spinach and mushroom mixture evenly among the chicken breasts, spooning it into the pocket you created. Over the filling, scatter the shredded mozzarella cheese.
- Securing the Chicken: Close the chicken breast over the filling and secure with toothpicks or kitchen twine to keep the filling from falling out during baking.
- Baking: Place the stuffed chicken breasts in the prepared

baking dish. Bake for 25 to 30 minutes in a preheated oven, or until the chicken is thoroughly cooked and its juices are clear.

- Serving: Once cooked, remove the toothpicks or twine before serving. Optionally, garnish with fresh herbs like parsley or basil for added flavor and presentation.

Time of Preparation

- Approximately 45 minutes.

Tips and Tricks

- If the chicken breasts are too thick, you can pound them gently with a meat mallet to even out the thickness, making it easier to stuff and cook evenly.
- Make sure the spinach and mushroom mixture is cooled slightly before stuffing the chicken to prevent the cheese from melting too quickly and leaking out.
- Experiment with different types of cheese for variation in flavor, such as feta or goat cheese.

Nutritional Value per Serving

Calories: 250 kcal

Protein: 30g

Fat: 10g

Carbohydrates: 5g

Fiber: 2g

Sugar: 2g

Caution and Precautions

- Use caution when handling raw chicken to prevent cross-contamination. After handling, properly wash your hands and any surfaces.
- Ensure the chicken reaches an internal temperature of at least 165°F (74°C) to ensure it is safe to eat.
- Remove toothpicks or twine carefully to avoid injury.

Health Benefits of this Recipe

- Lean protein, such that found in chicken, is necessary for the development and repair of muscles
- Spinach is packed with vitamins and minerals, including vitamin K, vitamin A, and folate, which are important for overall health and immunity.
- Mushrooms are low in calories and rich in antioxidants and fiber, which can aid in

- digestion and support a healthy gut.

Healthy Safety Measures

- Use fresh, high-quality ingredients to maximize nutritional value and minimize the risk of foodborne illnesses.

- Store leftovers in an airtight container in the refrigerator and consume within 2-3 days.
- Enjoy your delicious and nutritious Spinach and Mushroom Stuffed Chicken Breast!

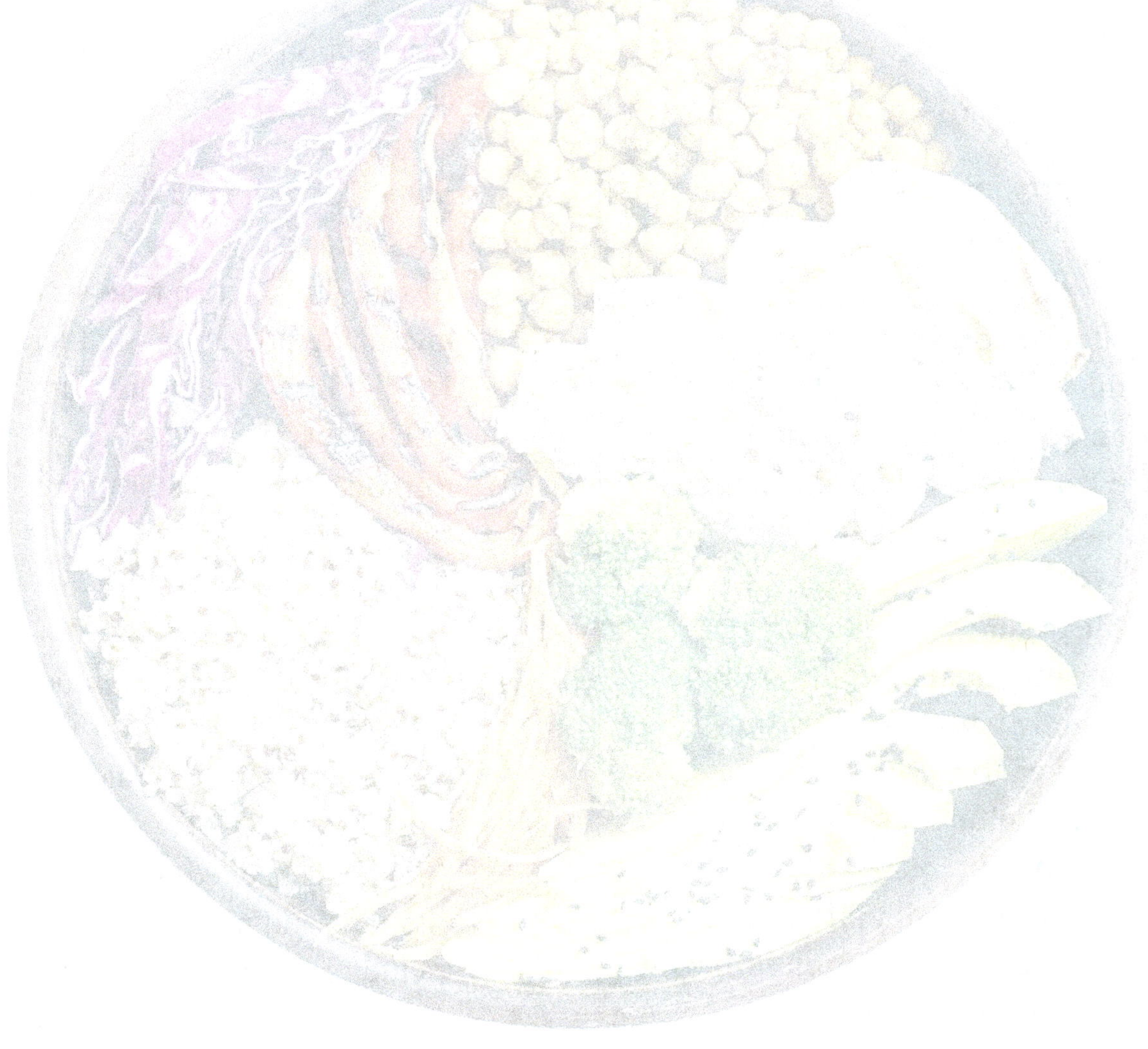

VEGETARIAN STIR-FRY WITH TOFU

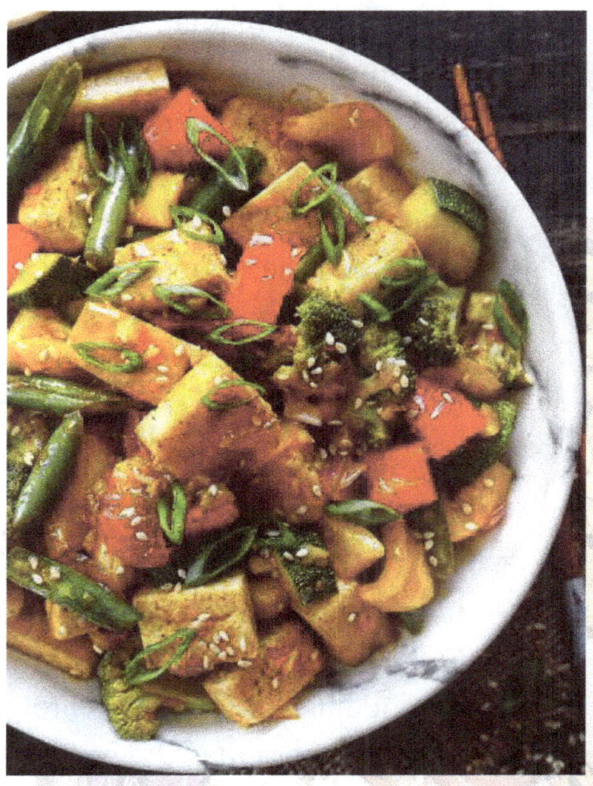

Ingredients

- Two cups of mixed veggies (such as bell peppers, broccoli, carrots, and snap peas) and one block (14 oz) of extra-firm tofu that has been pressed and cubed
- 3 tablespoons soy sauce
- 2 tablespoons hoisin sauce
- 1 tablespoon sesame oil
- 2 cloves garlic, minced
- 1 tablespoon grated ginger
- 2 green onions, chopped
- 2 tablespoons vegetable oil for stir-frying
- Cooked rice or noodles for serving

Procedure

- Tofu should first be pressed to eliminate any extra moisture. Place the tofu block between paper towels and place a heavy object on top, like a cast-iron skillet or a stack of plates. Let it press for at least 30 minutes, then cube the tofu.
- Marinade: In a small bowl, mix together soy sauce, hoisin sauce, sesame oil, minced garlic, grated ginger, and chopped green onions. Set aside.
- Stir-Frying: Heat vegetable oil in a large skillet or wok over medium-high heat. Add the cubed tofu and heat for 5 to 7 minutes, or until golden brown on all sides. Take out the tofu and place it aside in a skillet.
- Vegetables: In the same skillet, add more oil if needed and stir-fry the mixed vegetables until they are tender-crisp, about 5-7 minutes.
- Combine: Return the tofu to the skillet with the vegetables. Pour the marinade over the tofu and vegetables, tossing gently to coat everything evenly.Allow

the flavors to combine and the food to heat through for a further two to three minutes.

- Serving: Serve the vegetarian stir-fry over cooked rice or noodles. If desired, garnish with more finely chopped green onions or sesame seeds.

Time of Preparation

- Approximately 45 minutes.

Tips and Tricks

- For extra flavor, you can marinate the tofu in the sauce mixture for 30 minutes before cooking.
- Use a non-stick skillet or well-seasoned wok to prevent sticking and ensure even cooking.
- Don't overcrowd the skillet or wok when stir-frying to allow the vegetables to cook evenly and quickly.

Nutritional Value per Serving

- **Calories: 250 kcal**
- **Protein: 15g**
- **Fat: 12g**
- **Carbohydrates: 20g**
- **Fiber: 5g**
- **Sugar: 8g**

Caution and Precautions

- Be careful when pressing the tofu to avoid breaking or crumbling it.
- Use caution when handling hot oil and utensils during the stir-frying process to prevent burns.
- Ensure that the tofu is cooked thoroughly to avoid any risk of foodborne illness.

Health Benefits of this Recipe

- Tofu is a good source of plant-based protein and contains all nine essential amino acids.
- Vitamins, minerals, and antioxidants—all of which are vital for general health and wellbeing—are abundant in vegetables.
- This recipe is low in saturated fat and cholesterol, making it heart-healthy and suitable for those watching their cholesterol levels.

Healthy Safety Measures

- Use fresh vegetables and tofu from a reputable source to ensure quality and safety.
- Wash hands, utensils, and cutting boards thoroughly before and after handling raw

ingredients to prevent cross-contamination.

- Store leftovers in an airtight container in the refrigerator and consume within 2-3 days.

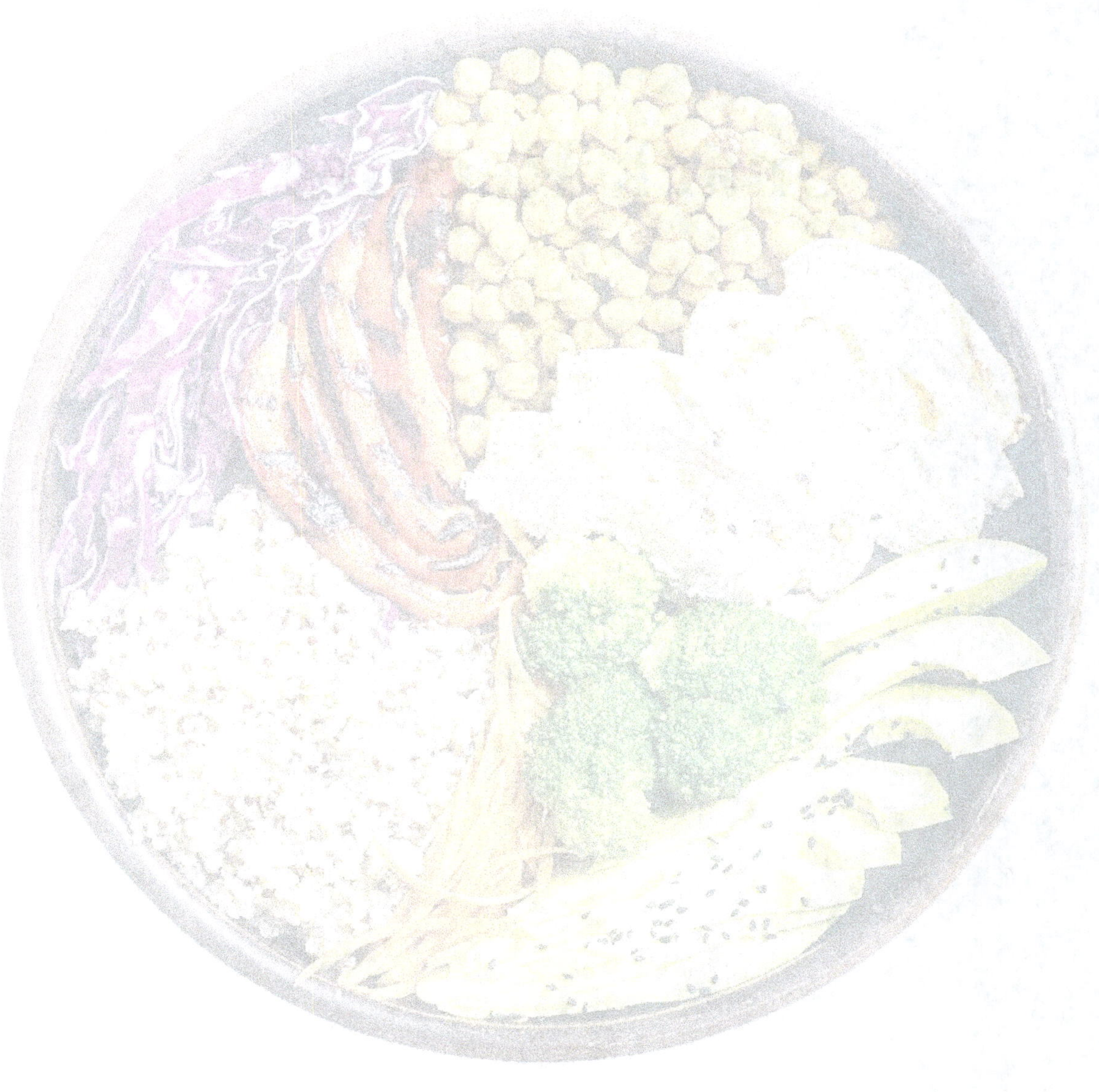

4

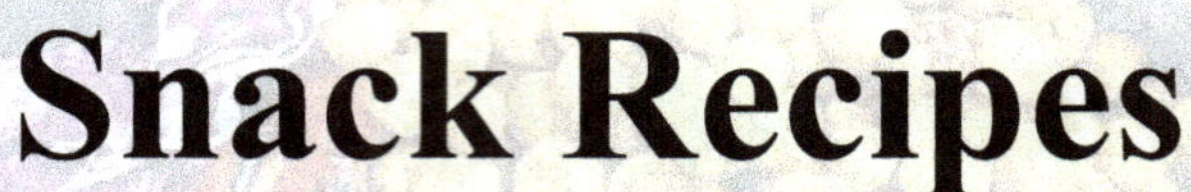

Snack Recipes

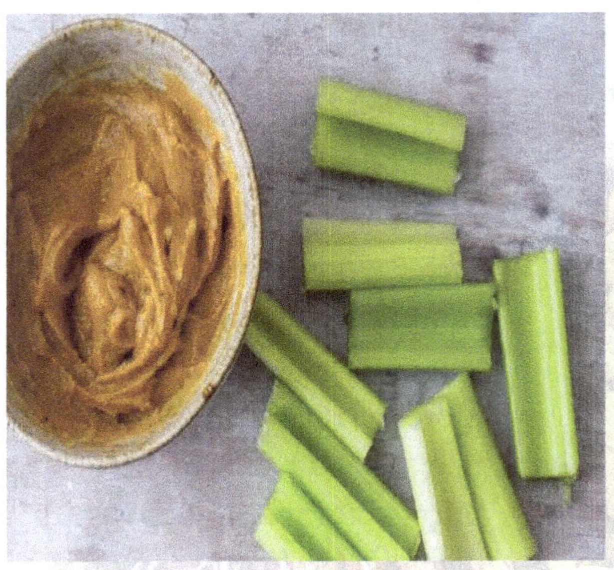

Ingredients

- Fresh celery stalks
- Almond butter (homemade or store-bought)
- Optional toppings: raisins, sliced almonds, chia seeds, shredded coconut

Procedure

- Wash the celery stalks thoroughly and pat them dry with a clean kitchen towel.
- Trim off the ends of the celery stalks and cut them into manageable-sized sticks, about 3-4 inches long.
- Spread a generous amount of almond butter along the concave side of each celery stick.
- Optionally, sprinkle your choice of toppings such as raisins, sliced almonds, chia seeds, or shredded coconut over the almond butter.
- Arrange the prepared celery sticks on a serving platter and serve immediately.

Time of Preparation

- Approximately 10 minutes

Tips and Tricks

- Ensure the celery stalks are fresh and crisp for the best texture.
- Try a variety of nut or seed butters to add some variation.
- For added crunch, lightly toast the sliced almonds before sprinkling them on top.
- Adjust the toppings to suit your diet or personal preferences.

Nutritional Value Per Serving (4 celery sticks with almond butter)

- **Calories: 120**

- **Total Fat: 9g**
- **Saturated Fat: 1g**
- **Cholesterol: 0mg**
- **Sodium: 80mg**
- **Total Carbohydrates: 7g**
- **Dietary Fiber: 3g**
- **Sugars: 2g**
- **Protein: 4g**

Caution and Precautions

- Check for nut allergies before serving almond butter to guests.
- Be cautious when serving to young children to prevent choking hazards.
- Any leftovers can be kept in the refrigerator for up to two days in an airtight container.

Health Benefits of This Recipe

- Celery is an excellent option for managing weight and maintaining digestive health because it is low in calories and high in fiber.
- Almond butter is a good source of healthy fats, protein, and vitamins, promoting heart health and providing sustained energy.
- The combination of celery and almond butter offers a satisfying snack that can help stabilize blood sugar levels and keep cravings at bay.
- Optional toppings like raisins and almonds add extra nutrients and antioxidants to the snack.

Healthy Safety Measures

- Wash hands thoroughly before handling ingredients.
- Use clean utensils and kitchen equipment to prevent contamination.
- Store perishable ingredients like almond butter in the refrigerator when not in use to maintain freshness.
- If preparing for a group, consider individual servings or portion control to prevent cross-contamination.

KALE CHIPS

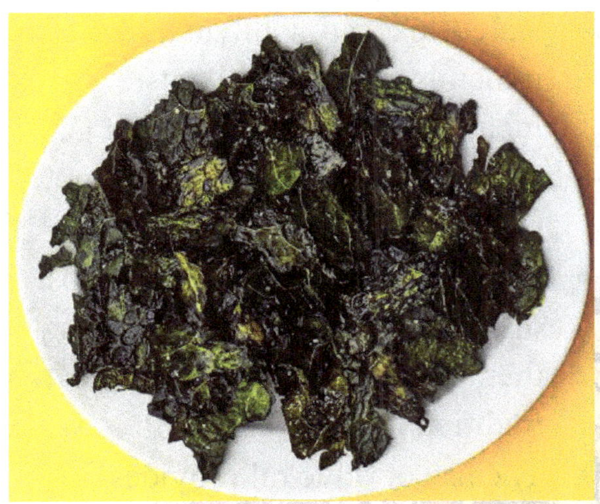

Ingredients

- Fresh kale leaves (preferably curly kale)
- Olive oil or avocado oil
- Salt (preferably sea salt or Himalayan salt)
- Optional seasonings: garlic powder, onion powder, paprika, nutritional yeast, or Parmesan cheese (for non-vegan option)

Procedure

- Before beginning, preheat the oven to 300°F (150°C) and place parchment paper on a baking sheet.
- Using paper towels or a salad spinner, thoroughly wash the kale leaves and pat dry.
- Tear the kale leaves into bite-sized pieces after removing the tough stems.
- In a large bowl, toss the kale pieces with olive oil, ensuring they are evenly coated but not drenched.
- Sprinkle salt and any desired seasonings over the kale, tossing again to distribute them evenly.
- Make sure the seasoned kale pieces do not overlap as you arrange them in a single layer on the baking sheet that has been prepared.
- Bake the kale chips for ten to fifteen minutes in a preheated oven, or until they are crisp but not burnt. They can turn from crispy to burnt very quickly, so keep an eye on them.
- Before serving, take the kale chips out of the oven and allow them to cool on the baking sheet for a few minutes

Time of Preparation

- Approximately 20 minutes

Tips and Tricks

- Use curly kale for the crispiest chips, as it holds up better to baking.

- Massage the oil into the kale leaves with your hands to ensure even coating and maximum crispiness.
- Find your favorite flavor combination by experimenting with different seasonings.
- Store any leftover kale chips in an airtight container at room temperature for up to 3 days.

Nutritional Value Per Serving (1 cup of kale chips)

- Calories: 50
- Total Fat: 3g
- Saturated Fat: 0g
- Cholesterol: 0mg
- Sodium: 200mg
- Total Carbohydrates: 6g
- Dietary Fiber: 1g
- Sugars: 1g
- Protein: 2g

Caution and Precautions

- Monitor the baking process closely to prevent the kale chips from burning.
- Be careful when handling hot baking sheets and kale chips straight out of the oven.
- Avoid overcrowding the baking sheet, as this can result in uneven cooking and soggy chips.

Health Benefits of This Recipe

- Kale is packed with vitamins, minerals, and antioxidants, including vitamin K, vitamin C, and beta-carotene, which promote overall health and wellbeing.
- Baking kale chips preserves most of their nutritional value, making them a healthier alternative to traditional potato chips.
- The use of olive oil provides healthy monounsaturated fats, which can help reduce inflammation and lower the risk of heart disease.
- Kale chips are naturally low in calories and carbohydrates, making them suitable for various dietary preferences and weight management goals.

Healthy Safety Measures

- Wash hands thoroughly before handling ingredients and utensils.
- Use clean kitchen equipment and surfaces to prevent contamination.
- Monitor the temperature of the oven to ensure even baking and avoid burning the kale chips.
- Store any leftover ingredients properly to maintain freshness and prevent spoilage.

BERRY YOGURT PARFAIT

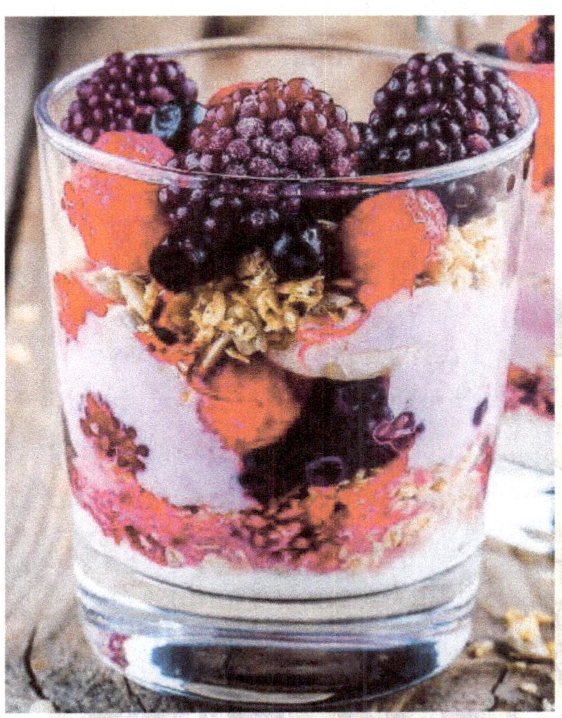

Ingredients

- Greek yogurt (plain or flavored)
- Mixed berries, such as strawberries, blueberries, raspberries, or blackberries, can be found either fresh or frozen.
- Granola (homemade or store-bought)
- Honey or maple syrup (optional, for sweetness)
- Optional toppings: sliced almonds, shredded coconut, chia seeds, or dark chocolate chips

Procedure

- If using frozen berries, thaw them in the refrigerator or microwave them briefly until they reach room temperature.
- In a serving glass or bowl, layer Greek yogurt, followed by a layer of mixed berries.
- Sprinkle a layer of granola over the berries, followed by another layer of yogurt.
- Repeat the layering process until the glass or bowl is filled, ending with a layer of yogurt on top.
- If you'd like, drizzle some honey or maple syrup on top of the yogurt layer for extra sweetness.
- Add optional garnishes like dark chocolate chips, chia seeds, shredded coconut, or sliced almonds.
- Serve immediately or store in the refrigerator until ready to eat.

Time of Preparation

- Approximately 10 minutes

Tips and Tricks

- Use Greek yogurt for a thicker consistency and higher protein content.
- Mix the yogurt with honey or maple syrup before layering to sweeten it evenly.
- Experiment with different combinations of berries and toppings to suit your taste preferences.
- For added crunch, toast the granola in the oven before layering it in the parfait.

Nutritional Value Per Serving

- **Calories: 250**
- **Total Fat: 7g**
- **Saturated Fat: 1g**
- **Cholesterol: 5mg**
- **Sodium: 50mg**
- **Total Carbohydrates: 35g**
- **Dietary Fiber: 5g**
- **Sugars: 20g**
- **Protein: 15g**

Caution and Precautions

- Check for any allergies to yogurt, berries, or nuts before serving to guests.
- Use caution when serving to young children to prevent choking hazards, especially with small toppings like nuts or chocolate chips.
- Any leftovers can be kept in the fridge for up to 1-2 days if they are kept in an airtight container.

Health Benefits of This Recipe

- Probiotics, which improve digestion and intestinal health, are abundant in Greek yogurt along with calcium and protein.
- Berries are packed with antioxidants, vitamins, and fiber, which promote overall health and immune function.
- Granola provides complex carbohydrates and fiber for sustained energy and improved digestion.
- The combination of yogurt, berries, and granola offers a balanced mix of macronutrients and micronutrients for a satisfying and nutritious snack or breakfast option.

Healthy Safety Measures

- Wash hands thoroughly before handling ingredients and serving utensils.
- Use clean bowls, glasses, and kitchen equipment to prevent contamination.

- If using fresh berries, wash them thoroughly under cold water and pat them dry with a clean kitchen towel.
- Store any perishable ingredients like yogurt and berries in the refrigerator until ready to use to maintain freshness and prevent spoilage
- .

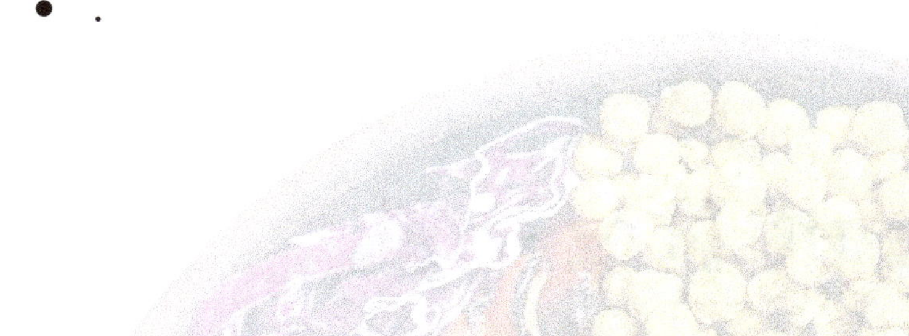

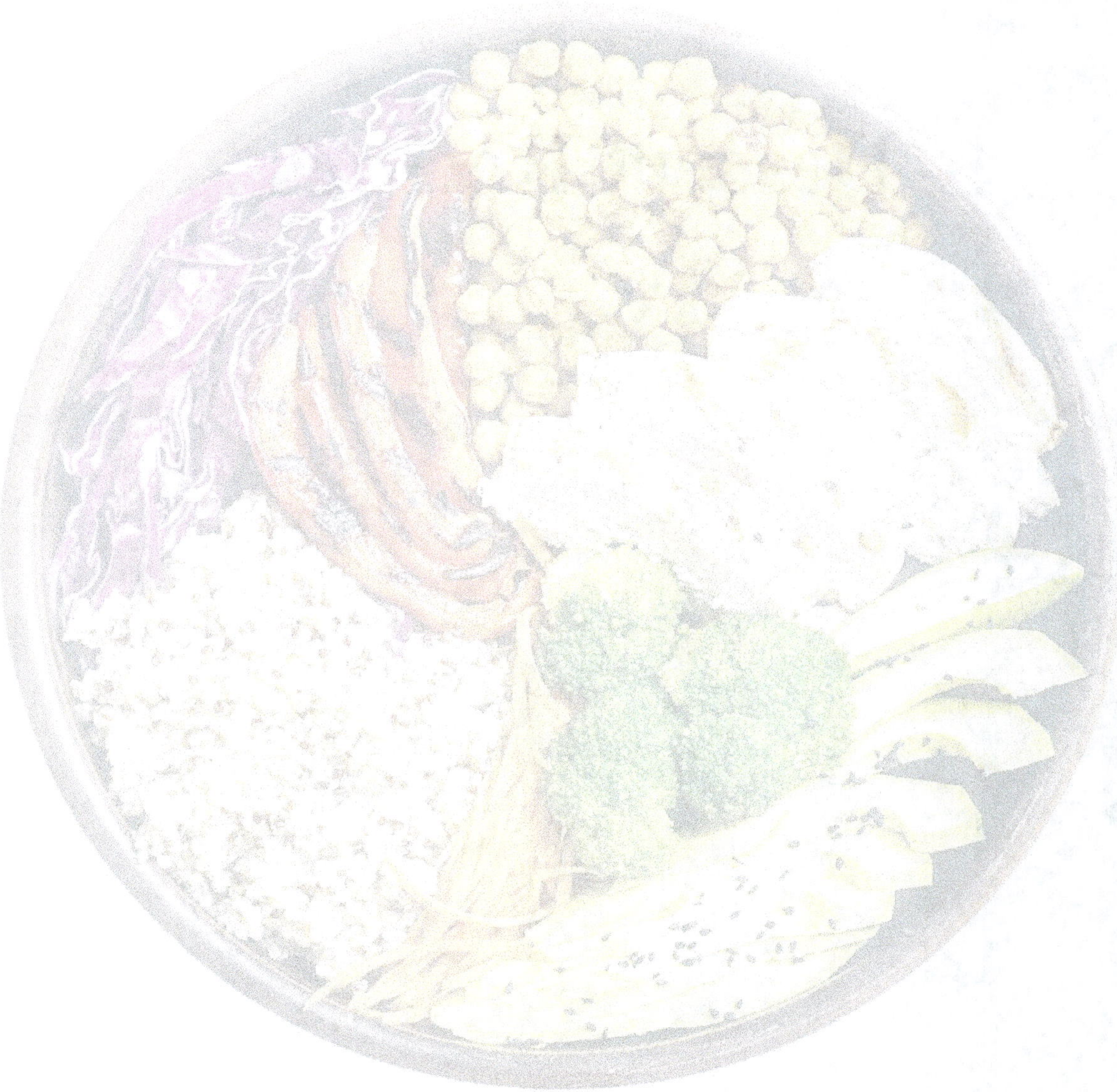

5

Dessert Recipes

CHIA SEED PUDDING

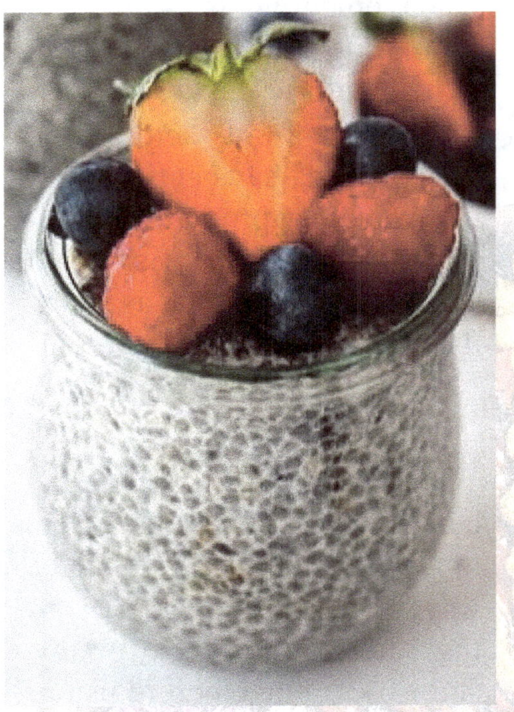

Ingredients

- 1/4 cup chia seeds
- One cup almond milk, or any other type of milk you prefer
- One tablespoon of optionally sweetened maple syrup or honey
- 1/2 teaspoon vanilla extract
- Fresh fruits (such as berries, banana slices, or mango chunks) for topping

Procedure

- In a mixing bowl, combine chia seeds, almond milk, honey or maple syrup (if using), and vanilla extract.
- To guarantee that the chia seeds are dispersed equally, thoroughly stir the mixture.
- To avoid clumping, whisk the mixture once more after letting it sit for about five minutes.
- To enable the chia seeds to absorb the liquid and take on the consistency of pudding, cover the bowl and place it in the refrigerator for at least two hours or overnight.
- Once chilled and set, stir the pudding again before serving to break up any clumps.
- Serve the chia seed pudding topped with fresh fruits of your choice.

Time of Preparation

- Approximately 2 hours (including chilling time)

Tips and Tricks

- Experiment with different types of milk (e.g., coconut milk, soy milk) to find your favorite flavor combination.
- To suit your taste, you can add more or less honey or maple syrup to change the sweetness level.
- For extra flavor, try adding a sprinkle of cinnamon or a dash of cocoa powder to the pudding mixture before chilling.

- Store any leftover chia seed pudding in an airtight container in the refrigerator for up to 3 days.

Nutritional Value per Serving (without toppings)

- **Calories: Approximately 120**
- **Fat: 6g**
- **Carbohydrates: 12g**
- **Fiber: 10g**
- **Protein: 4g**

Caution and Precautions

- If you have a history of digestive issues or are sensitive to high-fiber foods, start with a smaller serving size of chia seed pudding to avoid discomfort.
- Pregnant or nursing women should consult with a healthcare professional before incorporating chia seeds into their diet.

Health Benefits of this Recipe

- Chia seeds are rich in fiber, omega-3 fatty acids, antioxidants, and various nutrients, making them a nutritious addition to your diet.
- The high fiber content of chia seeds can promote digestive health and regularity, while also helping to control blood sugar levels and lower cholesterol.
- Consuming chia seed pudding as a healthy snack or breakfast option may help support weight management goals by promoting satiety and reducing overall calorie intake.
- The omega-3 fatty acids found in chia seeds have anti-inflammatory properties that may help reduce the risk of chronic diseases such as heart disease and arthritis.

Healthy Safety Measures

- Wash your hands thoroughly before handling any ingredients to prevent the spread of bacteria.
- Use fresh, high-quality ingredients, and check for any signs of spoilage before using.
- Store perishable ingredients such as almond milk in the refrigerator to maintain freshness.
- Clean and sanitize all utensils, bowls, and surfaces used during food preparation to prevent cross-contamination.

AVOCADO CHOCOLATE MOUSSE

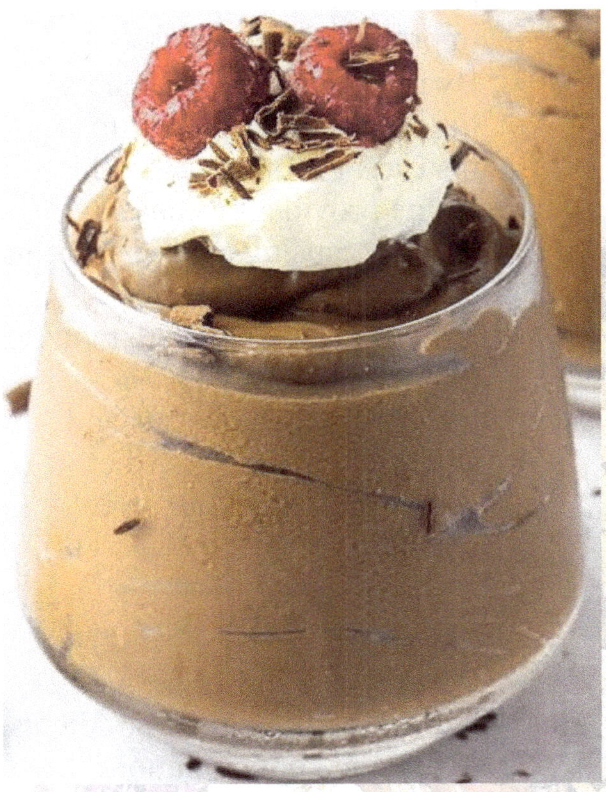

Ingredients

- 2 ripe avocados
- 1/4 cup cocoa powder
- 1/4 cup maple syrup or honey, or more according to taste
- 1 teaspoon vanilla extract
- Pinch of salt
- Optional garnishes include almond slices, coconut flakes, and fresh berries.

Procedure

- Halve the avocados, remove the pits, and transfer the flesh to a food processor or blender.
- Add cocoa powder, honey or maple syrup, vanilla extract, and a pinch of salt to the blender or food processor.
- Blend the mixture until smooth and creamy, scraping down the sides of the blender or food processor as needed to ensure all ingredients are well incorporated.
- If extra honey or maple syrup is needed, taste the mousse and adjust the sweetness.
- Once the desired consistency and sweetness are achieved, transfer the mousse to serving dishes or bowls.
- Before serving, let the food cool for at least half an hour in the refrigerator.
- If preferred, garnish with chopped almonds, coconut flakes, or fresh berries

Time of Preparation

- Approximately 15 minutes (excluding chilling time)

Tips and Tricks

- Make sure to use ripe avocados for the creamiest texture and best flavor.
- If you prefer a thicker mousse, add less honey or maple syrup. For a lighter mousse, you can add a splash of almond milk or coconut milk.
- Experiment with different toppings such as crushed nuts,

shaved chocolate, or a sprinkle of sea salt to enhance the flavor and presentation of the mousse.
- To make the mousse even smoother, you can strain it through a fine mesh sieve before chilling.

Nutritional Value per Serving

- **Calories: Approximately 200**
- **Fat: 15g**
- **Carbohydrates: 20g**
- **Fiber: 9g**
- **Protein: 3g**

Caution and Precautions

- While avocados are generally safe for most people, those with latex allergies may also be allergic to avocados.Be cautious if you have a history of allergies.
- Check the ripeness of avocados before using them. Overripe avocados may have a bitter taste and affect the overall flavor of the mousse.
- Any leftover mousse can be kept in the fridge for up to two days in an airtight container.Health

Benefits of this Recipe

- Avocados are some nutrient-dense fruit rich in heart-healthy monounsaturated fats, fiber, vitamins, and minerals.

- Cocoa powder is a good source of antioxidants and may help reduce inflammation and improve heart health.
- By using natural sweeteners like honey or maple syrup instead of refined sugar, this recipe provides sweetness without causing a rapid spike in blood sugar levels.
- This avocado chocolate mousse is a delicious way to incorporate healthy fats and antioxidants into your diet while satisfying your sweet cravings.

Healthy Safety Measures

- Wash your hands thoroughly before handling any ingredients to prevent contamination.
- Choose organic and pesticide-free avocados and cocoa powder whenever possible to minimize exposure to harmful chemicals.
- Clean all utensils, blender blades, and surfaces used during food preparation to prevent cross-contamination.

COCONUT MANGO SORBET

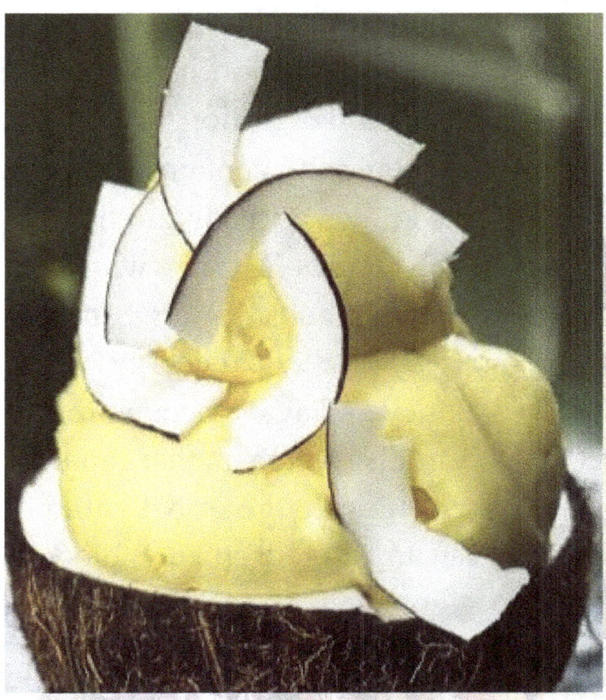

Ingredients

- 2 ripe mangoes, peeled and diced
- 1 can (13.5 oz) coconut milk
- Taste and adjust 1/4 cup agave nectar or honey.
- 1 tablespoon lime juice
- Optional: shredded coconut for garnish

Procedure

- Place the diced mangoes, coconut milk, honey or agave nectar, and lime juice in a blender or food processor.
- Blend the mixture until smooth and creamy.
- Taste the mixture and adjust sweetness if necessary by adding more honey or agave nectar.
- Transfer the blend onto a baking pan or shallow dish.
- Cover the dish or pan with plastic wrap and freeze for about 4-6 hours, or until firm.
- After the sorbet has frozen, take it out of the freezer and allow it to come to room temperature for a short while so that it can soften a little.
- Scoop the sorbet into serving bowls or cones, garnish with shredded coconut if desired, and serve immediately.

Time of Preparation

- Approximately 10 minutes (excluding freezing time)

Tips and Tricks

- For maximum sweetness and flavor, use ripe mangoes. In the event that fresh mangoes are unavailable, frozen mango chunks can be substituted.
- For a creamier texture, use full-fat coconut milk. Light coconut milk can be used for a lighter

option, but the texture may be slightly less creamy.

- Adding a splash of rum or coconut rum to the mixture before freezing can enhance the flavor and add a subtle tropical twist.
- To make the sorbet more refreshing, you can add a handful of fresh mint leaves to the blender along with the other ingredients.

Nutritional Value per Serving

- **Calories: Approximately 200**
- **Fat: 10g**
- **Carbohydrates: 28g**
- **Fiber: 3g**
- **Protein: 2g**

Caution and Precautions

- Check the consistency of the sorbet periodically while freezing. If it becomes too hard, you can let it soften at room temperature for a few minutes before serving.
- Be cautious when handling the blender or food processor to avoid injury.
- Store any leftover sorbet in an airtight container in the freezer for up to 1 week.

Health Benefits of this Recipe

- Mangoes are rich in vitamins A and C, antioxidants, and fiber, which can support immune health and digestion.
- Coconut milk contains healthy fats known as medium-chain triglycerides (MCTs), which may help boost metabolism and provide sustained energy.
- Honey and agave nectar are natural sweeteners that can add sweetness to the sorbet without causing a rapid spike in blood sugar levels.
- This coconut mango sorbet is a dairy-free and vegan-friendly dessert option that is lower in calories and fat compared to traditional ice cream.

Healthy Safety Measures

- Wash your hands thoroughly before handling any ingredients to prevent contamination.
- Use a clean blender or food processor and wash it well after use to prevent cross-contamination.
- Store any leftover sorbet in individual portions to make it easier to thaw and serve later.

LEMON GINGER DETOX WATER

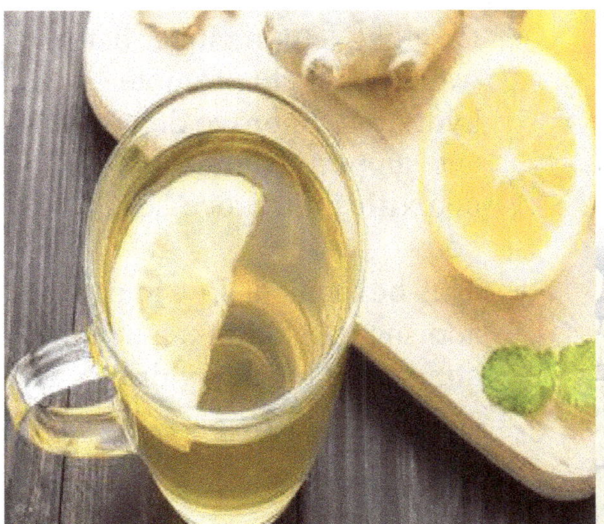

Ingredients

- 1 lemon, sliced
- 1-inch piece of ginger, sliced or grated
- 4-6 cups of water
- Optional: fresh mint leaves, cucumber slices, or a pinch of cayenne pepper for added flavor

Procedure

- Rinse the lemon and ginger under cold water to remove any dirt or debris.
- Cut the lemon into thin slices and peel the ginger if desired, then slice or grate it into small pieces.
- In a large pitcher, combine the lemon slices and ginger pieces.
- Add 4-6 cups of water to the pitcher, depending on how strong you want the flavor to be.
- Stir the mixture gently to distribute the lemon and ginger throughout the water.
- If desired, add fresh mint leaves, cucumber slices, or a pinch of cayenne pepper for additional flavor.
- Cover the pitcher and refrigerate for at least 1-2 hours to allow the flavors to infuse into the water.
- Serve the lemon ginger detox water chilled over ice.

Time of Preparation

- Approximately 5 minutes (excluding refrigeration time)

Tips and Tricks

- For a stronger flavor, you can squeeze the lemon slices slightly before adding them to the water to release more juice.
- To make the ginger flavor more intense, lightly crush the ginger slices with the back of a spoon before adding them to the pitcher.
- Experiment with different variations by adding other fruits such as oranges, grapefruits, or berries to the detox water.
- To make a larger batch, double or triple the ingredients and store the detox water in the refrigerator for up to 24 hours.

Nutritional Value per Serving

- **Calories: Approximately 10**
- **Fat: 0g**
- **Carbohydrates: 3g**
- **Fiber: 1g**
- **Protein: 0g**

Caution and Precautions

- Some people may be allergic to citrus fruits like lemons. If you experience any adverse reactions such as itching, swelling, or hives after consuming lemon detox water, discontinue use and consult a healthcare professional.
- Certain drugs or medical conditions may interact with ginger. If you have any concerns, consult with your healthcare provider before incorporating ginger into your diet.
- Pregnant or breastfeeding women should consult with a healthcare professional before consuming large amounts of ginger.

Health Benefits of this Recipe

- Lemon is a rich source of vitamin C and antioxidants, which can help boost immune function and support skin health.
- Ginger contains bioactive compounds such as gingerol, which have anti-inflammatory and antioxidant properties that may aid digestion and reduce nausea.
- Drinking lemon ginger detox water may help promote hydration, improve digestion, and support natural detoxification processes in the body.
- This beverage is low in calories and sugar, making it a healthy alternative to sugary drinks and sodas.

Healthy Safety Measures

- Wash your hands thoroughly before handling any ingredients to prevent contamination.
- Use filtered or purified water to ensure the best flavor and purity of the detox water.
- Clean the pitcher and utensils used for preparing the detox water with hot, soapy water to prevent bacterial growth.

CUCUMBER MINT COOLER

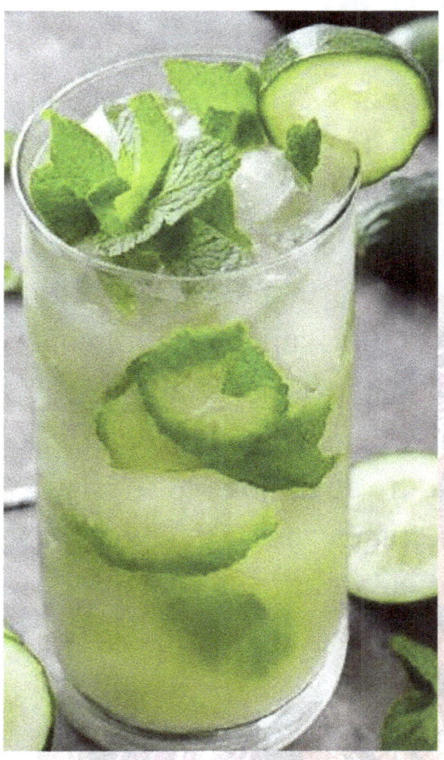

Ingredients

- 1 large cucumber, peeled and diced
- 1/4 cup fresh mint leaves
- 2 tablespoons lime juice
- 2 cups cold water
- Ice cubes
- Optional: honey or agave nectar to taste

Procedure

- In a blender, combine the diced cucumber, fresh mint leaves, lime juice, and cold water.
- Mix the ingredients until they are well blended and smooth.
- Taste the cooler and add honey or agave nectar if desired for sweetness, blending again to incorporate.
- Strain the mixture through a fine mesh sieve to remove any pulp or solids, if preferred.
- Pour the cucumber-mint concoction over the ice cubes that have been placed in glasses.
- Garnish each glass with a sprig of fresh mint or a slice of cucumber, if desired.
- Serve immediately and enjoy the refreshing cucumber mint cooler!

Time of Preparation

- Approximately 10 minutes

Tips and Tricks

- For a stronger mint flavor, lightly crush the mint leaves before adding them to the blender.
- To make the cooler extra refreshing, chill the glasses in the freezer before serving.
- You can customize the sweetness level of the cooler by adjusting the amount of honey

or agave nectar to suit your taste preferences.

- Try adding a splash of sparkling water or club soda for a fizzy variation of the cucumber mint cooler.

Nutritional Value per Serving

- **Calories: Approximately 25**
- **Fat: 0g**
- **Carbohydrates: 6g**
- **Fiber: 1g**
- **Protein: 1g**

Caution and Precautions

- Some individuals may be allergic to cucumbers or mint. If you experience any adverse reactions such as itching, swelling, or hives after consuming the cooler, discontinue use and consult a healthcare professional.
- Pregnant or breastfeeding women should consult with a healthcare professional before consuming large amounts of mint.

Health Benefits of this Recipe

- Cucumbers are low in calories and high in water content, making them a hydrating and refreshing addition to this cooler.
- Mint leaves contain menthol, which has a cooling effect and may help soothe digestive discomfort.
- Lime juice adds a burst of vitamin C and antioxidants to the cooler, supporting immune health and skin vitality.
- This cucumber mint cooler is a healthy alternative to sugary beverages, providing hydration and natural flavor without added sugars or artificial ingredients.

Healthy Safety Measures

- Wash your hands thoroughly before handling any ingredients to prevent contamination.
- Use fresh, high-quality ingredients and rinse the cucumber and mint leaves under cold water before use.
- Clean the blender and utensils used for preparing the cooler with hot, soapy water to prevent bacterial growth.
- Store any leftover cucumber mint cooler in the refrigerator in an airtight container for up to 2 days.

HERBAL INFUSIONS FOR LYMPHATIC HEALTH

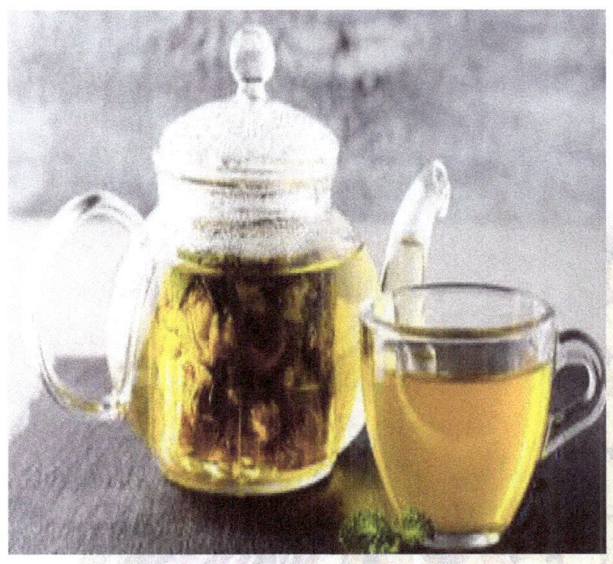

Ingredients

- 1 tablespoon dried red clover blossoms
- 1 tablespoon dried cleavers
- 1 tablespoon dried calendula flowers
- 4 cups hot water

Procedure

- Place the dried red clover blossoms, cleavers, and calendula flowers in a teapot or heatproof pitcher.
- Pour 4 cups of hot water over the herbs, covering them completely.
- Cover the teapot or pitcher with a lid or a plate and let the herbs steep for 10-15 minutes.
- After steeping, strain the herbal infusion through a fine mesh sieve or cheesecloth to remove the herbs.
- Pour the strained infusion into a mug or teacup and enjoy warm.

Time of Preparation

- Approximately 15 minutes

Tips and Tricks

- You can adjust the quantities of the herbs according to your taste preferences or availability.
- For a stronger infusion, allow the herbs to steep for a longer period of time, up to 30 minutes.
- Store any leftover herbal infusion in a sealed container in the refrigerator for up to 24 hours, and reheat before serving if desired.
- Add a squeeze of lemon juice or a drizzle of honey to enhance the flavor of the herbal infusion.

Nutritional Value per Serving

- **Calories: Approximately 5**
- **Fat: 0g**
- **Carbohydrates: 1g**
- **Fiber: 0g**
- **Protein: 0g**

Caution and Precautions

- Certain prescription drugs or medical problems may interact with certain plants. Consult with a healthcare professional before incorporating herbal infusions into your routine, especially if you are pregnant, breastfeeding, or taking medication.
- If you experience any adverse reactions such as allergic reactions or digestive upset after consuming herbal infusions, discontinue use and consult a healthcare professional.
- Ensure that the herbs used in the infusion are sourced from reputable suppliers and are free from contaminants.

Health Benefits of this Recipe

- Red clover blossoms are known for their potential lymphatic and blood-cleansing properties, helping to support lymphatic drainage and detoxification.
- Cleavers are traditionally used to promote lymphatic circulation and reduce swelling or congestion in the lymph nodes.
- Calendula flowers contain anti-inflammatory compounds that may help soothe lymphatic-related issues such as swollen lymph nodes or lymphedema.
- Consuming herbal infusions regularly as part of a balanced diet and healthy lifestyle may support overall lymphatic health and immune function.

Healthy Safety Measures

- Wash your hands thoroughly before handling any ingredients to prevent contamination.
- Use filtered or purified water to ensure the best flavor and purity of the herbal infusion.
- Clean the teapot or pitcher and any utensils used for preparing the infusion with hot, soapy water to prevent bacterial growth.
- Store any leftover herbal infusion in the refrigerator and consume within 24 hours to prevent spoilage.

6

Sauces and Dressings

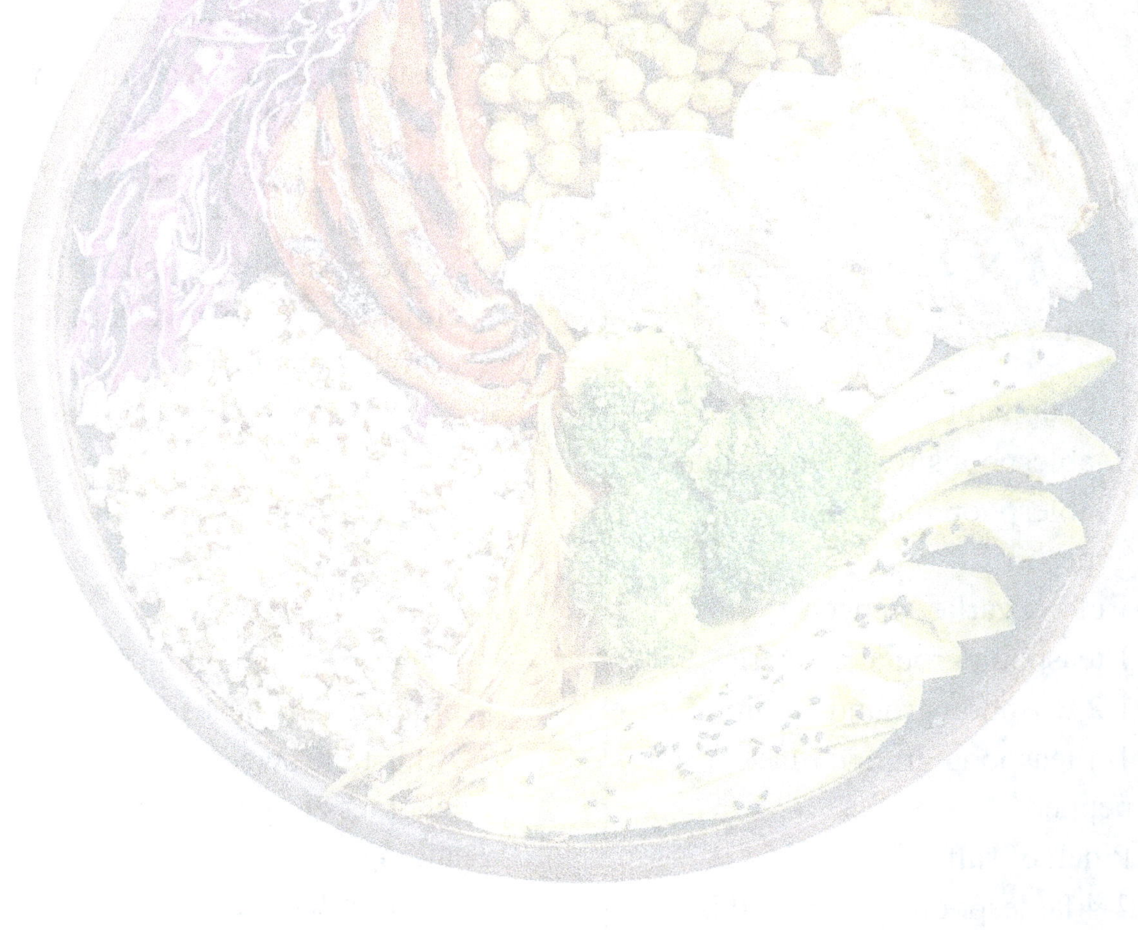

TURMERIC TAHINI DRESSING

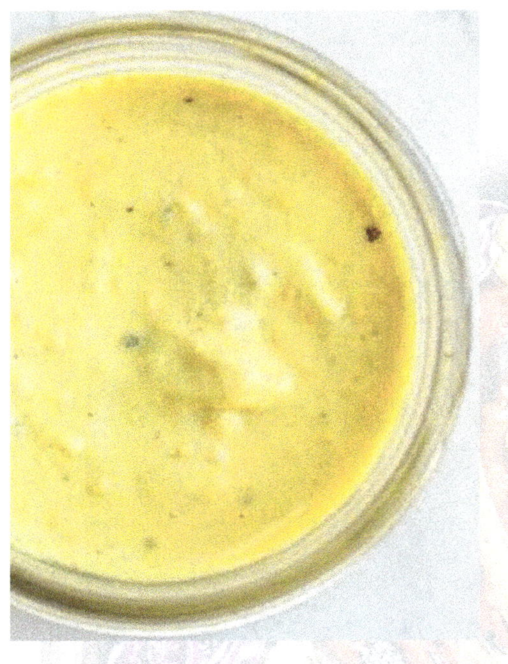

Ingredients

- 1/4 cup tahini
- 2 tablespoons fresh lemon juice
- 1 tablespoon maple syrup or honey
- 1 clove garlic, minced
- 1 teaspoon ground turmeric
- 1/2 teaspoon ground cumin
- 1/4 teaspoon ground black pepper
- Pinch of salt
- 2-4 tablespoons water, to thin as needed

Procedure

- In a small bowl, whisk together tahini, lemon juice, maple syrup or honey, minced garlic, ground turmeric, ground cumin, black pepper, and salt until well combined.
- One tablespoon at a time, gradually add water until the required consistency is achieved. The dressing needs to be pourable and creamy.
- Taste and adjust seasoning if necessary, adding more salt, lemon juice, or sweetener to taste.
- Serve right away or keep chilled for up to a week in an airtight container.

Time ofPreparation

- Approximately 10 minutes

Tips and Tricks

- Using fresh lemon juice produces the best flavor.
- Adjust the sweetness and tanginess to your preference by adding more or less maple syrup or lemon juice.
- If the tahini is too thick, microwave it for a few seconds

or stir vigorously to loosen it up before using.

- Feel free to customize the dressing by adding herbs like parsley or cilantro, or a pinch of cayenne pepper for extra heat.

Nutritional Value per Serving (1 tablespoon)

- **Calories: 45**
- **Total Fat: 3.5g**
- **Saturated Fat: 0.5g**
- **Sodium: 15mg**
- **Carbohydrates: 3g**
- **Fiber: 0.5g**
- **Sugars: 1g**
- **Protein: 1g**

Caution and Precautions

- Turmeric may stain clothing and countertops, so handle it carefully.
- If you have any allergies or sensitivities to sesame seeds (tahini), garlic, or any other ingredients, be cautious and adjust the recipe accordingly.
- Always use fresh and high-quality ingredients to ensure the best taste and nutritional value.

Health Benefits of this Recipe

- Turmeric contains curcumin, a compound known for its anti-inflammatory and antioxidant properties, which may help reduce inflammation and support overall health.
- Tahini is rich in healthy fats, protein, and vitamins and minerals like calcium and iron, which can contribute to heart health and bone strength.
- Garlic has antimicrobial properties and may help boost the immune system and promote cardiovascular health.

Healthy Safety Measures

- Both before and after handling ingredients, properly wash your hands.
- Maintain sanitized and clean surfaces to avoid cross-contamination.
- Store leftovers promptly in the refrigerator to prevent spoilage and foodborne illness.
- Use separate utensils and cutting boards for raw and cooked ingredients to avoid contamination.

BASIL PESTO SAUCE

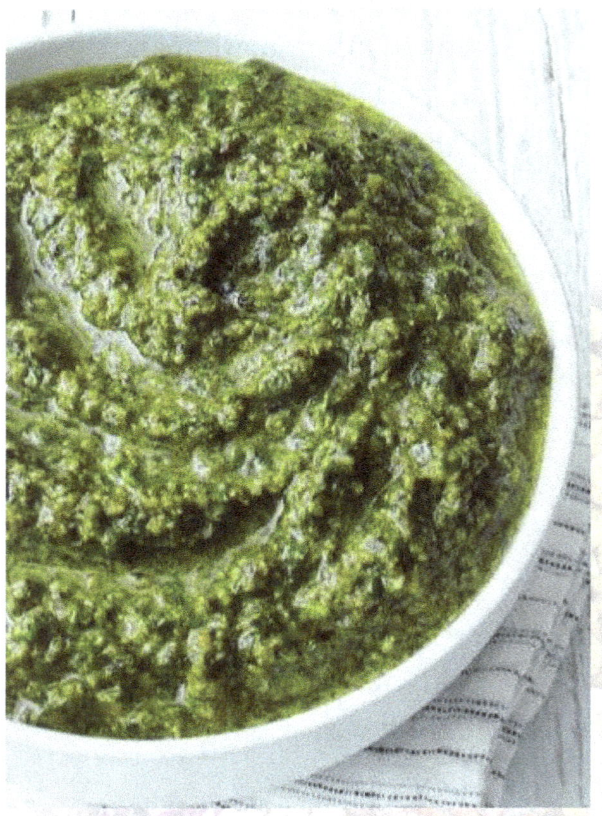

Ingredients

- 2 cups fresh basil leaves, packed
- 1/2 cup grated Parmesan cheese
- 1/2 cup extra virgin olive oil
- 1/3 cup pine nuts or walnuts
- 3 garlic cloves, minced
- Salt and pepper to taste

Procedure

- In a food processor or blender, combine basil leaves, Parmesan cheese, pine nuts or walnuts, and minced garlic.
- Once the ingredients are properly blended and coarsely chopped, pulse the mixture.
- Olive oil should be added gradually while the food processor is operating, until the pesto has the consistency you want. Periodically, you might need to pause and scrape down the bowl's sides.
- Season with salt and pepper to taste, and pulse again to incorporate.
- Taste and adjust seasoning if necessary.

Time of Preparation

- Approximately 15 minutes

Tips and Tricks

- The flavor of the nuts can be improved by toasting them before combining them with the pesto. Simply place them in a dry skillet over medium heat and cook, stirring frequently, until lightly browned and fragrant.
- If you prefer a smoother pesto, you can blanch the basil leaves in boiling water for 15-20 seconds, then immediately transfer them to an ice bath to

stop the cooking process before blending.

- For a nuttier flavor, try using roasted nuts instead of raw.
- Store-bought grated Parmesan cheese can be used, but freshly grated Parmesan will provide the best flavor.

Nutritional Value per Serving (2 tablespoons)

- **Calories: 140**
- **Total Fat: 14g**
- **Saturated Fat: 2g**
- **Cholesterol: 4mg**
- **Sodium: 100mg**
- **Carbohydrates: 1g**
- **Fiber: 0g**
- **Sugars: 0g**
- **Protein: 2g**

Caution and Precautions

- Be cautious when using a food processor or blender, and follow the manufacturer's instructions to avoid injury.
- If you have a nut allergy, you can omit the nuts or substitute them with sunflower seeds or pumpkin seeds.
- Store pesto in an airtight container in the refrigerator and use within one week, or freeze in ice cube trays for longer storage.

Health Benefits of this Recipe

- Basil is rich in vitamins A, K, and C, as well as antioxidants like flavonoids and polyphenols, which may help reduce inflammation and support immune health.
- A good source of monounsaturated fats that can lower cholesterol and lower the risk of heart disease is olive oil.
- Nuts are packed with protein, fiber, and essential nutrients like vitamin E and magnesium, which can support heart health and brain function.

Healthy Safety Measures

- Hands should be well cleaned both before and after handling ingredients.
- Use clean utensils and equipment to prevent contamination.
- Store leftovers properly to maintain freshness and prevent foodborne illness.
- Be mindful of allergens and dietary restrictions when serving pesto to guests.

CITRUS VINAIGRETTE

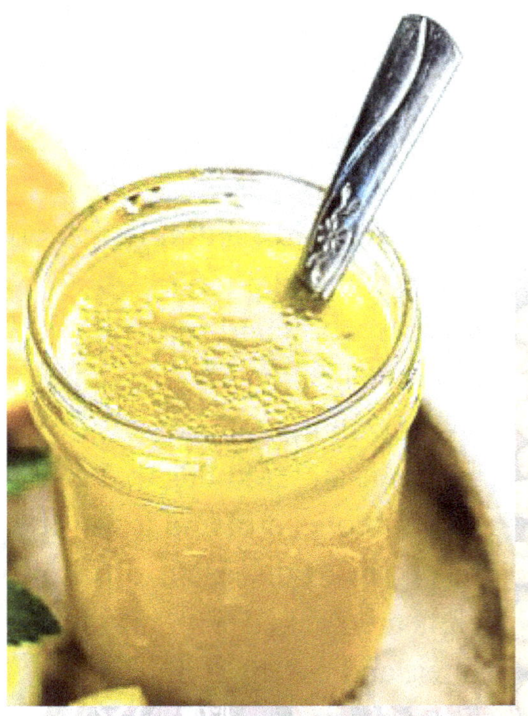

Ingredients

- 1/4 cup fresh orange juice
- 2 tablespoons fresh lemon juice
- 2 tablespoons white wine vinegar
- 1 teaspoon Dijon mustard
- 1 teaspoon honey or maple syrup
- 1/2 cup extra virgin olive oil
- Salt and pepper to taste

Procedure

- In a small bowl or jar, combine fresh orange juice, lemon juice, white wine vinegar, Dijon mustard, and honey or maple syrup.
- Whisk or shake vigorously until well combined.
- Slowly drizzle in the extra virgin olive oil while continuing to whisk or shake until the dressing is emulsified and smooth.
- Season with salt and pepper to taste.
- Taste and adjust seasoning if necessary.

Time of Preparation

- Approximately 5 minutes

Tips and Tricks

- For optimal flavor, use freshly squeezed lemon and orange juice.
- If you prefer a sweeter dressing, you can increase the amount of honey or maple syrup.
- For a more intense citrus flavor, you can add grated orange or lemon zest to the dressing.
- Experiment with different types of vinegar, such as champagne vinegar or apple cider vinegar, for unique flavor variations.

Nutritional Value per Serving (2 tablespoons)

- **Calories: 120**
- **Total Fat: 14g**
- **Saturated Fat: 2g**
- **Sodium: 20mg**
- **Carbohydrates: 2g**
- **Sugars: 1g**
- **Protein: 0g**

Caution and Precautions

- Be cautious when handling citrus fruits and sharp utensils to avoid injury.
- Check the expiration dates of the ingredients to ensure freshness.
- Store the vinaigrette in an airtight container in the refrigerator and use within one week.

Health Benefits of this Recipe

- Citrus fruits like oranges and lemons are rich in vitamin C, which can boost the immune system and promote skin health.
- Olive oil is high in monounsaturated fats, which can help reduce the risk of heart disease and inflammation.
- Honey or maple syrup provide natural sweetness and may have antibacterial and antioxidant properties.

Healthy Safety Measures

- Handle ingredients with clean hands both before and after.
- Use clean utensils and equipment to prevent contamination.
- Store leftovers properly to maintain freshness and prevent foodborne illness.
- Be mindful of any allergies or dietary restrictions when serving the vinaigrette to guests.

STEAMED BROCCOLI WITH GARLIC

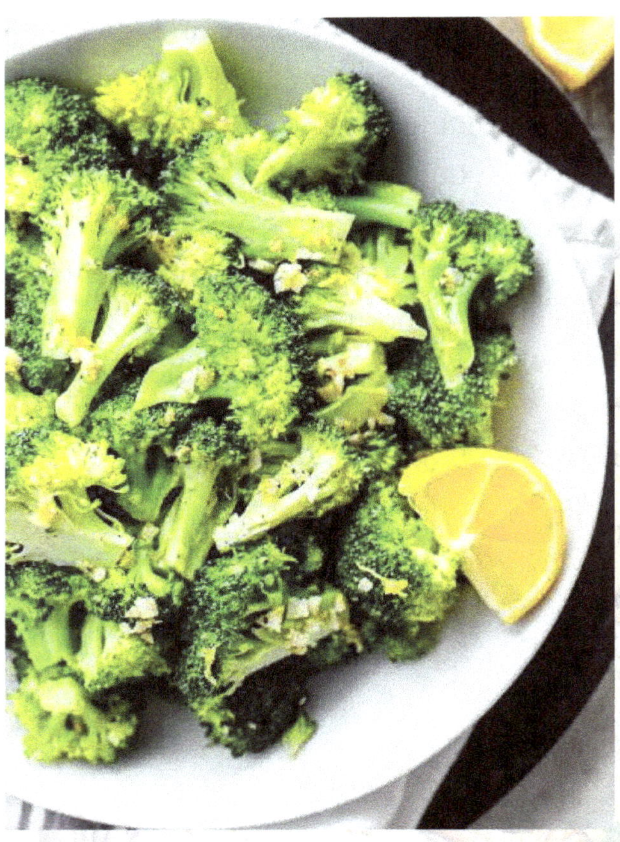

Ingredients

- 1 head of broccoli, cut into florets
- 2 cloves garlic, minced
- 2 tablespoons olive oil
- Salt and pepper to taste
- Lemon wedges for serving (optional)

Procedure

- Begin by preparing the broccoli. Use cold running water to give the broccoli a good wash, then pat dry with paper towels.
- Cut the broccoli into florets, ensuring they are all roughly the same size for even cooking.
- In a steamer basket or pot fitted with a steaming rack, bring water to a boil over medium-high heat.
- Once the water is boiling, add the broccoli florets to the steamer basket or rack. Cover and steam for 5-7 minutes, or until the broccoli is tender but still vibrant green.
- While the broccoli is steaming, heat olive oil in a small skillet over medium heat. Saute the minced garlic for one to two minutes, or until it becomes aromatic and slightly browned. Take off the heat.
- After the broccoli is done, move it to a platter. Drizzle the garlic-infused olive oil over the steamed broccoli and toss gently to coat.
- Season with salt and pepper to taste.If preferred, garnish the hot dish with lemon slices for extra freshness.

Time of Preparation

- Approximately 15-20 minutes

Tips and Tricks

- Don't overcook the broccoli; steaming it for too long can result in a mushy texture and loss of nutrients.
- For extra flavor, you can sprinkle grated Parmesan cheese or red pepper flakes over the steamed broccoli before serving.
- If you don't have a steamer basket, you can also steam the broccoli in a microwave-safe dish with a little water, covered with plastic wrap or a microwave-safe lid.

Nutritional Value per Serving

- **Calories: 80 kcal**
- **Protein: 3g**
- **Fat: 7g**
- **Carbohydrates: 4g**
- **Fiber: 2g**
- **Vitamin C: 80mg (133% DV)**
- **Vitamin K: 90mcg (113% DV)**

Caution and Precautions

- Be careful when removing the lid or plastic wrap from the steamed broccoli to avoid steam burns.
- Ensure the broccoli is thoroughly washed to remove any dirt or debris before cooking.

Health Benefits of This Recipe

- Broccoli is a nutrient-rich vegetable that is high in fiber, vitamins (such as vitamin C, vitamin K, and vitamin A), and minerals (such as potassium and calcium).
- Garlic contains compounds with potential health benefits, including anti-inflammatory and immune-boosting properties.
- Steaming the broccoli helps retain its nutrients better than boiling, preserving its health benefits.

Healthy Safety Measures

- Before handling any ingredients, properly wash your hands with soap and water.
- Use separate cutting boards and utensils for raw meat and vegetables to prevent cross-contamination.
- Ensure the broccoli is cooked to the recommended temperature of 135°F (57°C) to kill any potential bacteria.

QUINOA PILAF

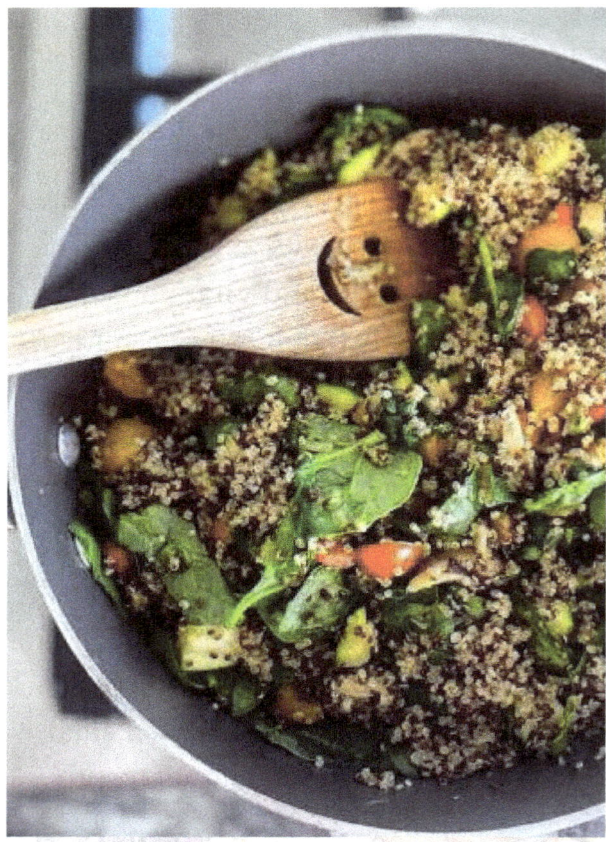

Ingredients

- 1 cup quinoa, rinsed thoroughly
- 2 cups vegetable broth or water
- 1 tablespoon olive oil
- 1 small onion, finely chopped
- 2 cloves garlic, minced
- 1 carrot, diced
- 1 bell pepper, diced
- 1/2 cup frozen peas
- 1 teaspoon dried thyme
- Salt and pepper to taste
- Fresh parsley for garnish (optional)

Procedure

- Heat the water or vegetable broth in a medium pot until it boils.
- Add the rinsed quinoa to the boiling broth, reduce the heat to low, cover, and simmer for about 15 minutes, or until the quinoa is tender and the liquid is absorbedTake it off the heat and leave it covered for five minutes.
- Heat the olive oil in a big skillet over medium heat while the quinoa cooks.
- Add the chopped onion and simmer for 3–4 minutes, or until transparent.
- Add the minced garlic, diced carrot, bell pepper, and frozen peas to the skillet. Cook for 5 to 7 minutes, stirring periodically, or until the vegetables are soft. Once the quinoa is cooked and fluffed with a fork, add it to the skillet with the cooked vegetables.
- Season with dried thyme, salt, and pepper to taste.
- Toss to ensure all the ingredients are well combined.
- If preferred, garnish with fresh parsley just before serving.

Time of Preparation

- Approximately 30 minutes

Tips and Tricks

- Rinse the quinoa thoroughly before cooking to remove its natural coating, called saponin, which can cause bitterness.
- For extra flavor, you can use vegetable broth instead of water to cook the quinoa.
- Feel free to customize the vegetables in the pilaf based on your preferences or what you have on hand.

Nutritional Value per Serving

- **Calories: 220 kcal**
- **Protein: 6g**
- **Fat: 6g**
- **Carbohydrates: 36g**
- **Fiber: 5g**

Caution and Precautions

- To prevent burns, exercise caution when working with hot liquids and steam.Ensure the quinoa is cooked thoroughly to avoid any risk of foodborne illness.

Health Benefits of This Recipe

- Quinoa is a gluten-free grain that is high in protein, fiber, and various vitamins and minerals, making it a nutritious alternative to rice or pasta.
- The vegetables in this pilaf provide essential nutrients such as vitamins A, C, and K, as well as antioxidants and fiber.
- Olive oil is a heart-healthy fat that contains monounsaturated fats and antioxidants.

Healthy Safety Measures

- Wash your hands and all vegetables thoroughly before cooking.
- Use separate cutting boards and utensils for raw meat and vegetables to prevent cross-contamination.
- Ensure leftovers are stored in the refrigerator within two hours of cooking to prevent bacterial growth.

ROASTED SWEET POTATOES

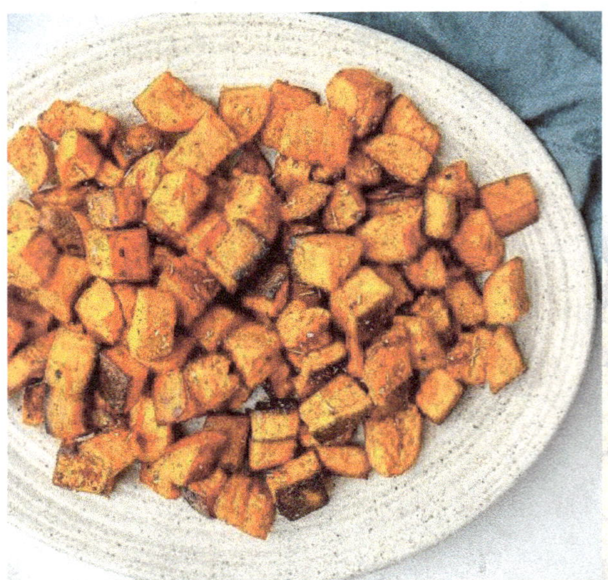

Ingredients

- Peel and chop two large sweet potatoes into pieces.
- 2 tablespoons olive oil
- 1 teaspoon paprika
- 1 teaspoon garlic powder
- 1 teaspoon dried thyme
- Salt and pepper to taste
- Fresh parsley for garnish (optional)

Procedure

- Adjust the oven temperature to 425°F (220°C) and place parchment paper or aluminum foil on a baking sheet.
- In a large bowl, toss the sweet potato cubes with olive oil, paprika, garlic powder, dried thyme, salt, and pepper until evenly coated.
- Arrange the seasoned sweet potatoes on the baking sheet that has been preheated in a single layer.
- Sweet potatoes should be roasted in a preheated oven for 25 to 30 minutes, or until they are soft and caramelized. Turn them halfway through to ensure equal browning.
- Once roasted, remove the sweet potatoes from the oven and transfer them to a serving dish.
- If desired, garnish before serving with fresh parsley.

Time of Preparation

- Approximately 35-40 minutes

Tips and Tricks

- Cut the sweet potato cubes into similar sizes to ensure even cooking.
- For extra crispiness, you can preheat the baking sheet in the oven before adding the sweet potatoes.
- Don't overcrowd the baking sheet; give the sweet potatoes some space to roast properly.

Nutritional Value per Serving

- **Calories: 150 kcal**
- **Protein: 2g**
- **Fat: 7g**
- **Carbohydrates: 20g**
- **Fiber: 4g**
- **Vitamin A: 400% DV**
- **Vitamin C: 4% DV**
- **Potassium: 15% DV**

Caution and Precautions

- Be careful when handling sharp knives and hot baking sheets to avoid cuts and burns.
- Make sure the sweet potatoes are cut into manageable sizes to prevent choking hazards, especially for young children.

Health Benefits of This Recipe

- Sweet potatoes are rich in beta-carotene, which is converted into vitamin A in the body, essential for vision health and immune function.
- The fiber in sweet potatoes promotes digestive health and helps regulate blood sugar levels.
- Olive oil used in this recipe provides heart-healthy monounsaturated fats and antioxidants.

Healthy Safety Measures

- Wash your hands and all utensils thoroughly before handling the sweet potatoes.
- To avoid cross-contamination, chop raw meat and veggies on different cutting boards.
- Store leftovers in an airtight container in the refrigerator to prevent bacterial growth.

7

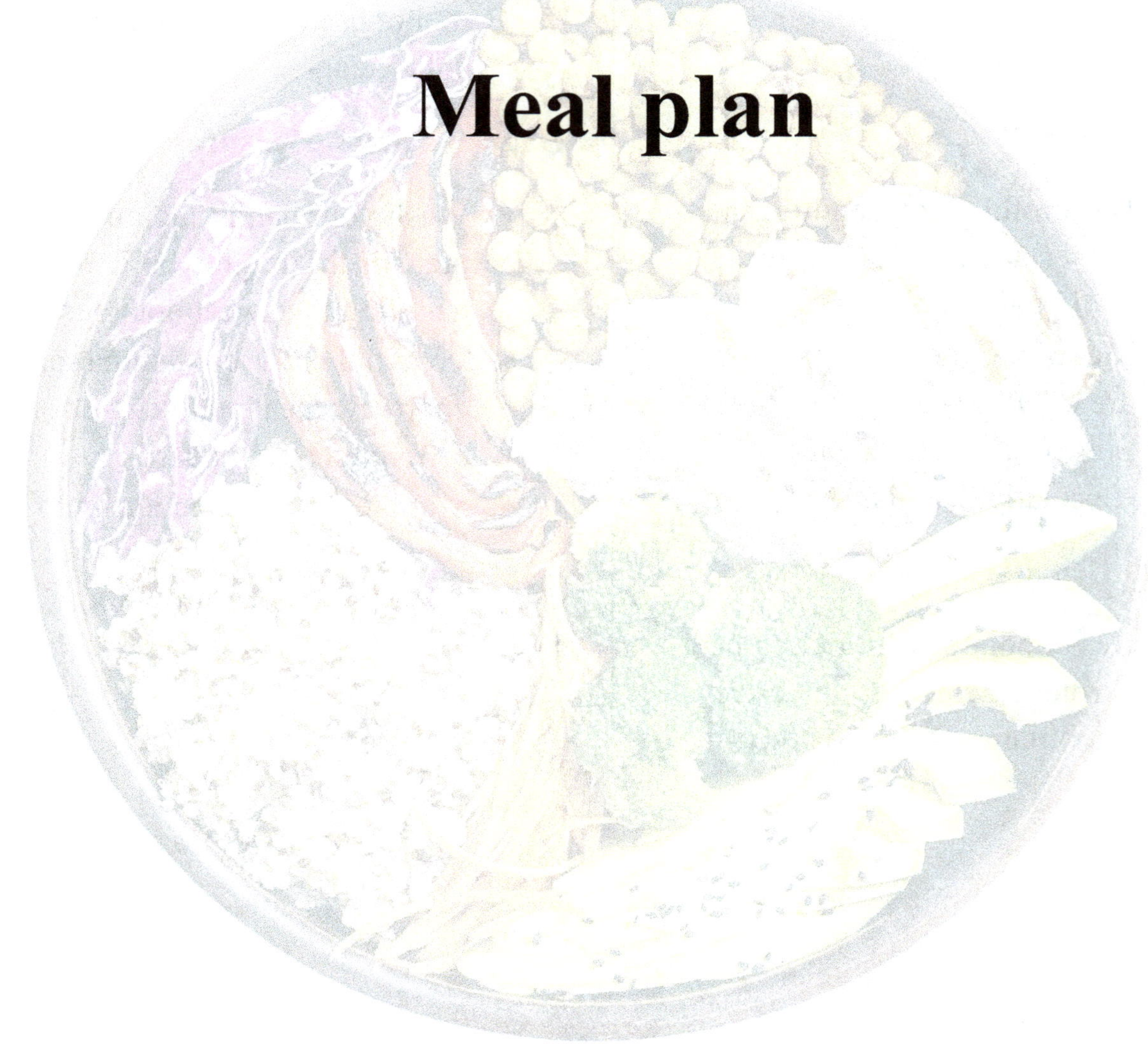

Meal plan

Day 1

- Breakfast: Lymphatic Boosting Smoothie
- Lunch: Lentil Soup with Turmeric
- Dinner: Grilled Vegetable Wrap

Day 2

- Breakfast: Quinoa Breakfast Bowl
- Lunch: Lymphatic Cleansing Salad
- Dinner: Garlic Ginger Salmon with Steamed Broccoli

Day 3

- Breakfast: Green Detox Juice
- Lunch: Spinach and Mushroom Stuffed Chicken Breast with Quinoa Pilaf
- Dinner: Vegetarian Stir-Fry with Tofu

Day 4

- Breakfast: Almond Butter Celery Sticks
- Lunch: Lentil Soup with Turmeric
- Dinner: Basil Pesto Grilled Vegetable Wrap

Day 5

- Breakfast: Kale Chips
- Lunch: Lymphatic Cleansing Salad
- Dinner: Garlic Ginger Salmon with Roasted Sweet Potatoes

Day 6

- Breakfast: Berry Yogurt Parfait
- Lunch: Lentil Soup with Turmeric
- Dinner: Vegetarian Stir-Fry with Tofu

Day 7

- Breakfast: Chia Seed Pudding
- Lunch: Spinach and Mushroom Stuffed Chicken Breast with Quinoa Pilaf
- Dinner: Green Detox Juice

Day 8

- Breakfast: Avocado Chocolate Mousse
- Lunch: Lymphatic Cleansing Salad
- Dinner: Grilled Vegetable Wrap

Day 9

- Breakfast: Coconut Mango Sorbet

- Lunch: Lentil Soup with
  Turmeric
- Dinner: Garlic Ginger Salmon
  with Steamed Broccoli

Day 10

- Breakfast: Lemon Ginger
  Detox Water
- Lunch: Spinach and Mushroom
  Stuffed Chicken Breast with
  Quinoa Pilaf
- Dinner: Vegetarian Stir-Fry
  with Tofu

Day 11

- Breakfast: Cucumber Mint
  Cooler
- Lunch: Lymphatic Cleansing
  Salad
- Dinner: Basil Pesto Grilled
  Vegetable Wrap

Day 12

- Breakfast: Herbal Infusions for
  Lymphatic Health
- Lunch: Lentil Soup with
  Turmeric
- Dinner: Garlic Ginger Salmon
  with Roasted Sweet Potatoes

Day 13

- Breakfast: Turmeric Tahini
  Dressing on Quinoa Breakfast
  Bowl

- Lunch: Spinach and Mushroom
  Stuffed Chicken Breast with
  Steamed Broccoli
- Dinner: Vegetarian Stir-Fry
  with Tofu

Day 14

- Breakfast: Citrus Vinaigrette on
  Lymphatic Boosting Smoothie
- Lunch: Lymphatic Cleansing
  Salad
- Dinner: Grilled Vegetable
  Wrap

Portion control guide

Lymphatic Boosting Smoothie

- Serving Size: 1 cup
- Portion Control: Enjoy one
  serving per serving time.

Quinoa Breakfast Bowl

- Serving Size: 1 bowl
- Portion Control: Serve one
  bowl per serving.

Green Detox Juice

- Serving Size: 1 glass (8 oz)

- Portion Control: Consume one glass per serving.

Lymphatic Cleansing Salad

- Serving Size: 1 plate
- Portion Control: One plate per serving.

Lentil Soup with Turmeric

- Serving Size: 1 bowl
- Portion Control: Serve one bowl per serving.

Grilled Vegetable Wrap

- Serving Size: 1 wrap
- Portion Control: Enjoy one wrap per serving.

Garlic Ginger Salmon

- Serving Size: 1 fillet
- Portion Control: Serve one fillet per serving.

Spinach and Mushroom Stuffed Chicken Breast

- Serving Size: 1 stuffed breast
- Portion Control: Serve one stuffed breast per serving.

Vegetarian Stir-Fry with Tofu

- Serving Size: 1 plate
- Portion Control: One plate per serving.

Almond Butter Celery Sticks

- Serving Size: 4 sticks
- Portion Control: Consume four sticks per serving.

Kale Chips

- Serving Size: 1 cup
- Portion Control: Enjoy one cup per serving.

Berry Yogurt Parfait

- Serving Size: 1 cup
- Portion Control: Serve one cup per serving.

Chia Seed Pudding

- Serving Size: 1 cup
- Portion Control: Enjoy one cup per serving.

Avocado Chocolate Mousse

- Serving Size: 1 cup
- Portion Control: Consume one cup per serving.

Coconut Mango Sorbet

- Serving Size: 1 scoop
- Portion Control: Serve one scoop per serving.

Lemon Ginger Detox Water

- Serving Size: 1 glass (8 oz)
- Portion Control: Consume one glass per serving.

Cucumber Mint Cooler

- Serving Size: 1 glass (8 oz)
- Portion Control: Enjoy one glass per serving.

Herbal Infusions for Lymphatic Health

- Serving Size: 1 cup
- Portion Control: Serve one cup per serving.

Turmeric Tahini Dressing

- Serving Size: 2 tablespoons
- Portion Control: Use two tablespoons per serving.

Basil Pesto Sauce

- Serving Size: 2 tablespoons
- Portion Control: Use two tablespoons per serving.

Citrus Vinaigrette

- Serving Size: 2 tablespoons
- Portion Control: Use two tablespoons per serving.

Sides and Accompaniments

- Steamed Broccoli with Garlic: Serve one cup per serving.
- Quinoa Pilaf: Serve one cup per serving.
- Roasted Sweet Potatoes: Serve one cup per serving.

CONCLUSION

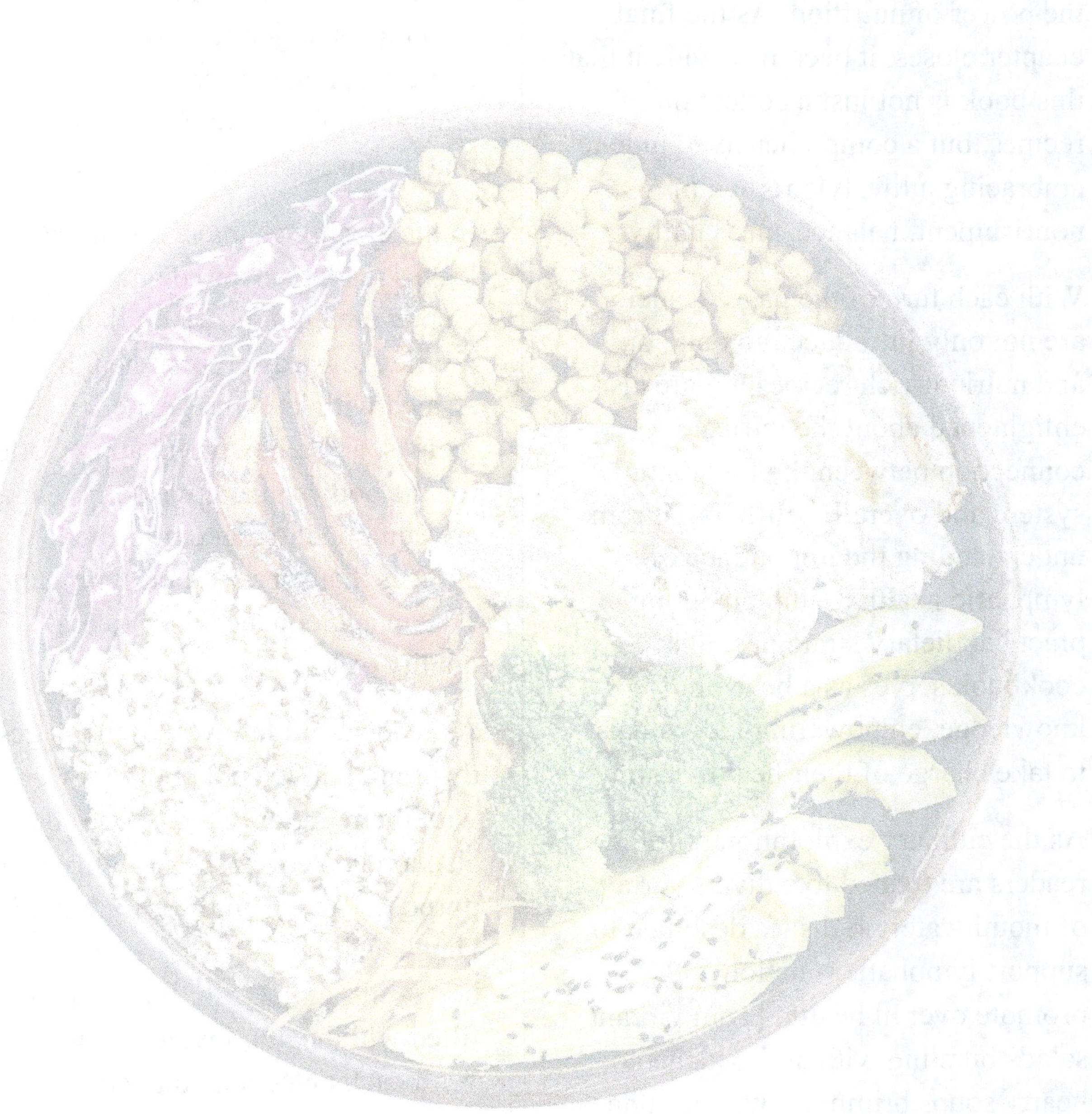

CONCLUSION

A transformative journey towards optimal health and wellness through the power of nutrition. As the final chapter closes, it becomes evident that this book is not just a collection of recipes, but a comprehensive guide to embracing a lifestyle rooted in nourishment, balance, and vitality.

With each turn of the page, readers are not only introduced to delicious and nutrient-rich recipes but are also enlightened about the intricate connection between the lymphatic system and overall well-being. From understanding the importance of lymphatic health to implementing practical dietary strategies, this cookbook serves as a beacon of knowledge, empowering individuals to take charge of their health destiny.

As the culinary exploration unfolds, readers are treated to a diverse array of mouthwatering dishes designed to support lymphatic function and promote overall health. From vibrant salads bursting with antioxidants to hearty soups brimming with immune-boosting ingredients, each recipe is crafted with care and intention, making every meal a celebration of wellness.

Beyond the kitchen, "The Complete Lymphatic Diet Cookbook" offers invaluable insights into lifestyle practices that complement dietary efforts. From stress management techniques to gentle movement exercises, readers are encouraged to embrace holistic wellness practices that nurture both body and soul.

In the closing chapters, the author leaves readers inspired and empowered to embark on their own journey towards optimal health. Armed with knowledge, delicious recipes, and a newfound appreciation for the body's innate wisdom, readers are equipped to make informed choices that support their lymphatic system and enhance their overall quality of life.

As readers bid farewell to the pages of this remarkable cookbook, they carry with them not only the recipes but also a renewed sense of vitality and purpose. "The Complete Lymphatic Diet Cookbook" is more than just a book—it's a blueprint for living a life filled with health, joy, and abundance. With each delectable bite and mindful practice, readers are reminded that true wellness begins from within, and the journey to vibrant health is as beautiful as it is delicious.

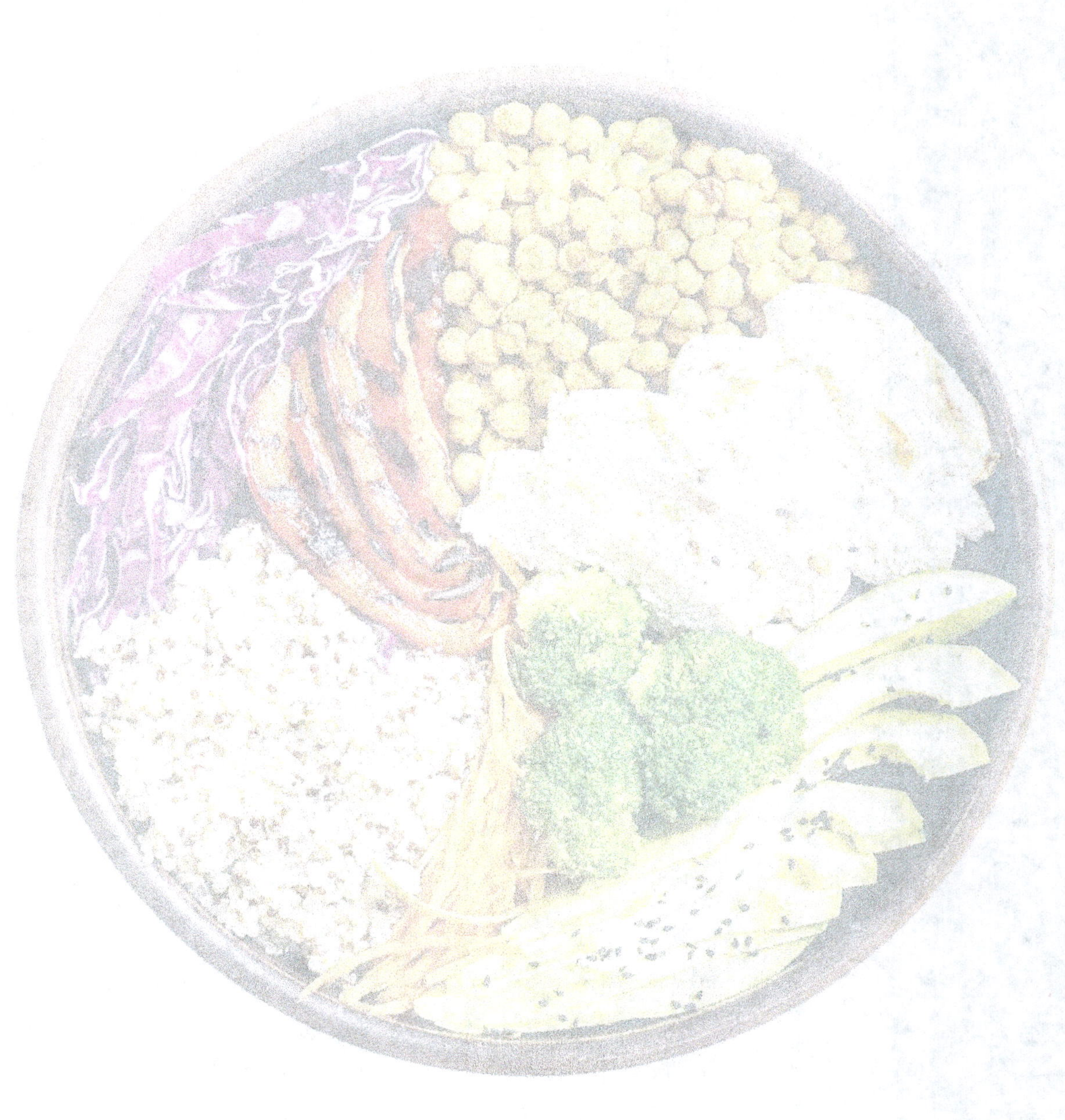